rejuvenation secrets from around the world

— that "work"!

Other books by Dr. Paavo Airola:

HOW TO GET WELL
ARE YOU CONFUSED?
THERE IS A CURE FOR ARTHRITIS
HEALTH SECRETS FROM EUROPE
CANCER: CAUSES, PREVENTION AND TREATMENT
          THE TOTAL APPROACH
STOP HAIR LOSS
SWEDISH BEAUTY SECRETS
SEX AND NUTRITION
HOW TO KEEP SLIM, HEALTHY, AND YOUNG
    WITH JUICE FASTING
THE MIRACLE OF GARLIC
EVERYWOMAN'S BOOK

Rejuvenation secrets from around the world

—that "work"!

Proven and effective ways to stop premature aging, and
live younger longer — by a world-famous authority

by Paavo O. Airola, N.D., Ph.D

HEALTH PLUS, Publishers
P. O. Box 22001, Phoenix, Arizona 85028

COPYRIGHT © 1974, BY

PAAVO O. AIROLA

ISBN 0-932090-09-5

FIRST PRINTING, JANUARY, 1974
SECOND PRINTING, NOVEMBER, 1975
THIRD PRINTING, DECEMBER, 1977
FOURTH PRINTING, MAY, 1980
FIFTH PRINTING, JUNE, 1981

Printed in the United States of America

Table of Contents

Dedication

The real purpose of attaining better physical health and a long life is not just mere enjoyment of life, but a higher, divine purpose for which life was given to us. All endeavors toward attaining better health and extended longevity would be a wasted effort unless the healthy body is used as a worthy temple for the spirit to dwell in and develop. The purpose of our lives is not just the building of magnificent bodies, or living a long time, but perfecting and refining our divine spirits, and becoming more God-like. Although this book deals with physical aspects of attaining an optimum level of health and long life, I wish to emphasize the divine nature and purpose of all life, and that the real purpose of achieving good health is to prepare a way for our spiritual growth, and refinement and perfection of our human and divine characteristics.

With these words, I dedicate this book *TO YOU*, sincerely hoping that it will not only help to improve your health and rejuvenate your body and mind, but also bring more happiness and purpose into your life.

Paavo O. Airola

Introduction

THE GREAT AMERICAN
YOUTH-QUAKE

We are living in the most exciting era of man's history. Headlines with world-shattering events are an every day occurrance. Age-long traditions are broken and discarded, and totally new values are formed. The pace of living is accelerated to an unprecedented tempo, and man's relation, not only to his fellow man, but also to his total environment, is undergoing dramatic changes. When the final history of mankind is written, the twentieth century will be known by many descriptive names. My humble contribution to the long list of fitting epithets includes: "The Epoch of Misguided Scientific Progress" . . . "The Slow-Extinction-Through-Chemistry Era" . . . "The Era of the High Protein Cult" . . . Gestapo Era of the FDA" . . . "The Age of Unholy Alliance Between Science and Food-Drug-Chemical Industries". But perhaps the most appropriate description of all for the second half of the twentieth century will be: "The Adulation-of-Youth Age" or "The Great American Youth-Quake".

Modern men and women are searching unrelentingly for ways and means to prolong youth and prevent the aging processes. Interest in methods of preventing premature aging and staying younger longer has never been as keen as it is at the present time. Hundreds of books are written on this subject. Diets, drugs, hormones, wraps, gadgets, tricks, face lifts, face peels, masks, herbs, cellular injections, cosmetic surgery, etc., are developed to fill the growing demand for the preservation or restoration of youth. Plastic surgeons and youth doctors make fortunes on the "adulation-of-youth" fad. We are going to great lengths in our efforts to prevent aging, and not only to *feel*, but also to *look* younger.

Even our modern science is engaged in a search for ways to prolong man's life and prevent the diseases and symptoms of aging. A special branch of medical science, gerontology, is busy working in research centers around the world to solve the secrets of aging and find ways of prolonging life. Some startling discoveries have been made in various parts of the world, but especially in Russia, Japan, Germany, and the United States. I will share with you in this book some of these discoveries in the art of staying young.

Of course, the search for secrets of rejuvenation and eternal youth is not a new phenomenon. Man has sought the fountain of youth since the dawn of history. Records from early medical history show a variety of herbs and foods used to retard the aging processes and revitalize aging bodies. The Papyrus of Eber, the oldest medical document known; the Hindu doctor, Susrata, 1400 B.C.; Chinese doctors of the third century – all recorded a significant interest in rejuvenation and offer various rejuvenation tonics.

However, human history has never known such a wide interest in rejuvenation as we have today. So many youth seekers are searching for the ways and means to slow up, halt, and even reverse the aging processes and preserve youth, that we are witnessing a rapid growth of a new kind of doctor – the so-called Youth Doctor – to satisfy the growing demand.

Unfortunately, the wide interest in rejuvenation has resulted in a correspondingly growing number of fake and quack rejuvenation methods and therapies. Gullible youth-seekers are being duped, exploited, and relieved of large sums of money, in return for which they receive worthless rejuvenative treatments, drugs, or injections.

To make this book as short and concise as possible, I will not waste your time by describing various unproven theories, or controversial treatments and drugs. I will report to you only *what is absolutely certain, solidly proven, and scientifically confirmed* – or, as the title promises, I will reveal to you rejuvenation secrets from around the world **THAT "WORK"**.

In my travels and studies in many countries around the world, I have found that natives have used for thousands of years certain herbs or natural foods and food substances to attain their good health and long life. For example, in a recent interview, the Mir (King) of Hunza said that the people of Hunza attribute their exceptional health and longevity to drinking their naturally hard (heavily mineralized) water. Thousands of years of actual application has demonstrated to the natives of Hunza that natural minerals in their water are helping to keep them in excellent health and to give them a long life. Recent scientific studies have shown that natural minerals in drinking water do have a decisive effect on man's health, and can help to prevent many killing diseases, such as heart disease, diabetes, and osteoporosis. In Russia, scientists have discovered that the diet of almost all of their centenarians is rich in natural, raw, unprocessed honey, which is heavily "contaminated" by pollen. In Finland, natives consider their hot saunas absolutely necessary to enjoy good health, prevent diseases, and prolong life. Modern science has confirmed that periodic artifically-induced fever, the kind the sauna bath creates, has a very beneficial effect on general metabolic process, and it helps to fight many diseases, including arthritis and cancer — and, thus, prolongs life.

In Mexico, scientists have discovered that a certain commonly used herb contains natural male and female sex hormones that can prevent senility and aging processes due to diminished hormone production, which is common with approaching old age.

Let's, therefore, examine these health and rejuvenation secrets from around the world that really "work" — secrets that are empirically proven — that is, proven by thousands of years of actual application.

1

REJUVENATION SECRETS
FROM
SWEDEN

Swedish women have long been known for their exceptional beauty, well-proportioned bodies, and luscious complexions, which they enjoy into advanced age. Sweden, a little Scandinavian country, has produced more internationally known beauties for the glamorous world of entertainment, and the Swedish girls have won more Miss World and Miss Universe titles than any other nation. Likewise, Swedish men are tall, handsome, and athletic. Sweden has one of the best health records in the world — the lowest infant mortality rate, and the highest life expentancy of any nation. This in spite of the fact that Sweden has one of the most rugged and unfriendly climates in the world, with large parts of it being located above the Polar Circle.

I have spent many years living in Sweden, and have made extensive studies of Swedish mode of living and their nutritional habits. I came to the conclusion that the exceptional health and beauty of the Swedish people are not unrelated phenomena, but are closely related to certain elements in their daily diet.

ROSE HIPS – SWEDISH HEALTH AND REJUVENATION SECRET NUMBER ONE!

The health and rejuvenative porperties of vitamin C have been recently confirmed by many scientific studies in Russia and the United States. Rose hips are the richest natural source of vitamin C, with the possible exception of acerola cherries. Russians call them "vitamin roses." Rose hips contain twenty to forty times more vitamin C than oranges! They are also rich in bioflavonoids, or vitamin P, and many other vitamins and minerals. Here's how rose hips compare with oranges:

- They have 28% more calcium.
- They have 25% more iron.
- They have 25 *times* more vitamin A!
- They have 20-40 times (depending on the variety) more vitamin C.

Rose hips have been introduced to the health-conscious world relatively recently – as a popular health food fad. But in Sweden, rose hips have been used very extensively for centuries! In fact, rose hips have always formed an essential part of the traditional Swedish diet. Swedes make nutritious soups, delicious vitamin-rich teas, jellies, and desserts from them. In Sweden, rose hips positively do not have the aura of a fad food about them. *All* Swedes use rose hips. They are sold in various forms in *all* food stores – not only health food stores – and are a staple food in the humble cottage as well as in the King's castle.

Because of the generous use of rose hips, the traditional Swedish diet has always been extremely rich in high quality natural vitamin C. Long before vitamin C was discovered, the Swedes, guided by natural instinct, gorged on rose hips, thus saturating their diet with vitamin C, *this health and rejuvenation vitamin number one.*

Rose hips grow wild in Sweden, especially in the northern parts of the country, where there are wide areas covered with bushes from which "hips" are picked in the fall. For the benefit of those who do not know, rose hips are the small (about the size of a cherry), fully ripened orange-red fruits just below the rose flower. Only certain varieties of rose bushes are suitable for eating. The best fruit-bearing varieties with the richest content of vitamin C are: Rosa Villosa, Rosa Canina, and Rosa Rugosa.

Collagen – key to perpetual youth.

Why are rose hips so important for health and long life? The latest scientific discoveries (by Drs. J. W. McCormick,

Johan Bjorksten, Roger Williams, and others) have shown that the aging processes and the degenerative changes of the skin — wrinkles, flabbiness, discoloration, etc. — are caused by physiological changes in collagen, the intercellular cement, which holds all the cells and tissues of the body together. Deterioration is caused primarily by a deficiency of vitamin C in the tissues. Sufficient vitamin C in the diet will keep collagen strong and elastic, which will result in tight skin and a smooth and lovely complexion.

Collagen is responsible for the stability and tensile strength of practically all of the tissues of the body, including the skin, the muscles, and the tissues of all organs and glands. The deficiency of vitamin C brings about the breakdown of this intercellular cement, and as a result of this, the instability and fragility of tissues. A vitamin C deficiency, in addition to adversely affecting your health in many other ways, will make your skin loose and flabby, saggy and lifeless, because of a loss of tension and elasticity. Wrinkles will appear early in life, eyes will lose their lustre, lips their fullness.

There are, of course, many other factors involved in feeding and maintaining a healthy skin, as we will see later in the book. Vitamins A, B-complex, minerals, and essential fatty acids are all important. But the breakdown of collagen, caused by a deficiency of vitamin C, is the main cause of the deterioration processes of the skin, and the primary contributing cause of premature aging.

When you finish reading this book, you will understand that the *secret of staying young is basically the secret of staying healthy,* and vitamin C plays a leading role in helping you to stay healthy, preventing disease, and extending your life in youthful vitality.

How vitamin C can keep you young.

Russian scientists have discovered that vitamin C has a profoundly stimulating effect on the adrenal glands. The adrenal glands secrete over 20 steroid hormones, which are directly involved in keeping your vital bodily processes in a condition of high efficiency. It is generally agreed that a decrease in the output of these hormones – which usually begins in late middle life – is responsible for the symptoms of aging. Russian scientists have demonstrated that substantial daily doses of vitamin C have a rejuvenative, stimulating effect on the glandular activity, and the hormones are once again produced in the higher levels, similar to those found in younger people.

The world-famous Nobel Prize Winner, Dr. Linus Pauling, reported that large doses of vitamin C may be effective in increasing male virility. It is a commonly known fact that potency and virility have been steadily declining during the last few decades, particularly in the United States. It is also a well-known fact that we have a grand scale vitamin C deficiency in the United States. The U. S. Department of Agriculture reports that 48% of all Americans have diets deficient in vital nutritive elements. Vitamin C was found to be one of the substances most lacking in the American diet. "Of the thousands of chemical tests on human adults to determine the body level of vitamin C, 90% were found deficient," said one of the world's leading vitamin C authorities, Dr. J. W. McCormick.

The healthy function of sex glands is directly related to the general health, and to the prolonged feeling and appearance of youth. The first signs of aging usually appear when sex hormone production begins to slow down. A Japanese doctor, M. Higuchi, has demonstrated that there is a relationship between vitamin C levels and the hormone production of the sex glands – the more vitamin C in the diet, the more sex hormones are produced by the glands. Prostatic fluid, which nourishes the sperm and keeps them alive, is extremely rich in vitamin C. A prolonged deficiency in vitamin C can slow down the hormone production of the sex glands and consequently contribute to premature aging.

Furthermore, there is a growing body of evidence that the aging process is largely a matter of the diminished oxygenation of cells. Vitamin C has a great effect on improved cell breathing, and, thus, can help prevent premature aging.

Hardening of the arteries, atherosclerosis, and heart attacks are true diseases of premature aging. Many doctors believe that "you are as old as your arteries." Boris Sokoloff, M. D., Director of the Southern Bio-Research Institute in Florida, reported that their conclusions, based on research and wide-spread evidence from medical literature, is that ascorbic acid (vitamin C) is the key factor in averting atherosclerosis, and, thus, preventing heart disease, our number one killer.

German professor, Werner Grab, M. D., has stated that vitamin C not only has curative powers in such diseases as hepatitis, influenza, rheumatic diseases, polio, metabolic diseases, and acute poisonings, but that even cancer will be inhibited by huge doses of ascorbic acid.

Vitamin C — the true fountain of youth!

If there ever has been a true miracle rejuvenative substance, vitamin C is it. It has so many universal applications that it is virtually impossible to find a condition of ill health or diminished well-being which vitamin C would not affect favorably, very often with a miraculous healing effect. Since old age is often associated with various conditions of diminished health, it stands to reason that vitamin C should be rejuvenative tonic number one for anyone over 40 years of age.

Vitamin C is completely non-toxic, and can be used in large doses — up to 10,000 to 20,000 mg. a day during short periods, or up to 5,000 mg. a day on a regular basis. A natural form of vitamin C, such as rose hips, is preferable, as it is accompanied by other vitamins of the C-complex, such as hesperidin, rutin, citrin, etc., which are generally called bioflavonoids. Bioflavonoids act as synergists with vitamin C, increasing its effect and making it biologically more potent.

WHEY — SWEDISH REJUVENATION SECRET NUMBER TWO

Whey is the liquid left over when cheese is made from milk. When the milk coagulates, the solid part — curds — is removed and the remaining liquid is called whey. In the United States, whey is usually thrown away or sold as a by-product for animal feed. In Sweden, whey is never wasted;

in fact, it is a national food. It is dehydrated and made into whey cheese (mesost) and whey butter (messmör).

In earlier times, when the Swedish dairy was neither industrialized nor mechanized, whey cheese and whey butter were made directly on the farms. Liquid whey was boiled in large iron kettles over the fire until the water evaporated, and the semi-solid whey remained. Then the whey was put into cloth or wooden forms to harden into cheese-like shapes and consistency — whey cheese. It was also put into glass jars and mixed with cream to form a butter-like spread — whey butter. Even now, in some parts of Sweden, Norway and Finland, whey cheese and whey butter are made by the farm women in this way. However, today the bulk of all whey products in Sweden is made in modern dairy factories by a modern evaporating process.

Colonic hygiene — secret of eternal youth.

Here are some scientific reasons why I consider whey to be an important health and rejuvenative factor in the Swedish diet.

Of all the "secrets" of perpetual youth, which man has uncovered and tried in his long search, none is more scientifically established than one which is based on the premise that *colonic hygiene* — or the perfectly and efficiently functioning digestive, assimilative and eliminative system — is the real secret of eternal youth.

Ilja Metchnikoff, the eminent Russian bacteriologist, made revolutionary discoveries at the turn of the century in regard to ways of prolonging life. He believed that auto-toxemia (self-poisoning) through putrefaction of metabolic wastes in the large intestine was the main cause of premature aging.

Your intestines house billions of bacteria which help your digestive system to break down the food you eat, and, thus, aid in the digestion and assimilation of nutrients. Many important nutrients, including some of the B-vitamins, are produced in the intestines by these intestinal bacteria. For optimum health, it is extremely important that there is always a plentiful supply of these beneficial bacteria.

Metchnikoff discovered that soured milks, and such milk products as whey, help feed the acidophilus and bifidus bacteria in the intestines and prevent the development of harmful putrefactive bacteria which lead to auto-toxemia. The more beneficial bacteria present in the colon, the less toxins produced by the putrefactive bacteria. Whey, which contains lactose, is the best natural food for these bacteria.

Thus, whey is perhaps the best food for preventing self-poisoning due to intestinal putrefaction, intestinal sluggishness, and constipation. Whey can also aid in the assimilation of nutrients from the foods you eat.

Constipation — enemy of health and longevity.

Many scientists believe that chronic intestinal sluggishness and constipation, together with faulty nutrition and poor digestion and assimilation of food, are the major contributing factors to many, if not most, illnesses and premature aging. The toxins, or poisons created by bacterial metabolism and putrefaction, remain in the intestines, and, as a result of prolonged constipation, are absorbed into the blood and, consequently, poison the whole organism. Thus, constipation can be directly linked to many rheumatic and arthritic conditions, eczema, and other skin disorders, bad breath, chronic headaches, nervous conditions, digestive disorders, colitis, and diverticulitis.

Whey is 77% lactose, which is a natural food for the friendly acidophilus and bifidus bacteria in the intestines. It has been scientifically established that using whey regularly will prevent constipation, internal sluggishness, gas, and bowel putrefaction.

Constipation is a number one enemy of beauty, too. A woman with a serious constipation problem can be spotted instantly; her skin has a muddy, gray tone; it is rough, porous, and often covered with eczema, pimples, and other blemishes; her breath is foul because her abused body is trying to purify its blood through the lungs. This was well understood by Cleopatra, famous for her clear, velvety, un-blemished and lusciously fresh complexion. According to Cleopatra's historian, Estelle Erlan, Cleopatra's "beauty secret" was her regular cleansing of the system with the mildly laxative leaves of *senna* to prevent constipation and keep her intesinal tract clean.

Swedish women — and men — keep their complexions unblemished, clear, and healthy with whey. By preventing constipation and cultivating beneficial vitamin-producing and disease-fighting bacteria in the intestines, whey also helps the Swedish people to enjoy excellent health and a longer life in youthful vitality.

In Sweden, whey is eaten daily by everyone. It is sold in all food stores, and you can find it on the table in every Swedish home in the form of cheese or butter.

In addition to being a miraculous cleanser and helping beneficial intestinal bacteria, whey is also an excellent food. It is rich in minerals, particularly iron, and vitamins, especially the age-fighting vitamin B_1. Here are a few nutritional facts about Swedish whey cheese:

- 77% of it is pure lactose — the active factor in its favorable influence on the intestinal tract.
- It has only 3.6% butter fat, as compared to 25% - 40% for ordinary cheese.
- It has 6 times more iron than beef, twice as much as beans or eggs, and 50% more than liver!
- It has 10 times more vitamin B_1 than ordinary cheese, twice as much as beef, and 5 times as much as milk.
- It has 7 times as much vitamin B_2 as beef, 20 times as much as milk, and 20 times as much as whole wheat flour.

Next to brewer's yeast, whey is the richest natural source of B_1 and B_2; these B-vitamins are extremely important for preserving a youthful appearance and preventing premature aging.

Unfortunately, whey cheese and whey butter are difficult to obtain in the United States. I have been successful in buying some in better cheese and delicatessen shops. *Whey powder* or *whey tablets*, sold in every health food store in the United States, are excellent substitutes for whey cheese and butter, having roughly the same nutritive and therapeutic value.

Make sure to incorporate whey into your diet, especially if you are prone to intestinal sluggishness, gas, or constipation. One or two tablespoons of whey powder a day, mixed with drinks or foods, is the suggested dose. Remember, whey -- the health and rejuvenative secret from Sweden — is not a drug, it is a natural miracle food which can help you to stay younger longer.

2

REJUVENATION SECRETS
FROM
FINLAND

The great, ancient physician, Parmenides, said two thousand years ago:

"Give me a chance to create fever, and I will cure any disease."

Two giants of modern medicine in Germany, Professor Werner Zabel, M.D., and Dr. Josef Issels, M.D., say:

"Artificially induced fever has the greatest potential in the treatment of many diseases, including cancer."

Med. Prof. Zabel told the following true story:

Until a few decades ago, the great Pontine swamps, not far from Rome, Italy, presented a constant source of malaria infections. Then, by government action, the swamps were dried out and malaria disappeared. But a remarkably strange observation was made recently. While earlier the whole malaria-infected area was free from cancer, now, a generation later, the population there shows the same incidence rate of cancer as the rest of Italy.

Dr. Zabel says that the mystery of the Pontine swamps has a simple solution: the frequent fever attacks, common in malaria patients, stimulated the body's own defenses so that cancer could not develop. Even when cancer had already developed, the exposure to malaria and the accompanying attacks of high fever had a curative effect on cancer.

It has also been reported from Italy, that there has never been observed any case of cancer on the Island of Sardinia, where practically everyone is affected by malaria.

Fever — misunderstood symptom

Fever has been too long a misunderstood and mistreated symptom. Most medical doctors try to combat and suppress fever. They see fever as a negative pathological condition which must be eliminated as fast as possible. With many modern fever-suppressing drugs, they quickly bring the fever down to "normal".

But things are beginning to change, and modern medical sicence is discovering (re-discovering) the therapeutic value of fever. Particularly in Europe, many biological clinics now use artificially induced fever to treat many of our most common diseases, including cancer. Famous French virologist and Nobel Prize Winner, Dr. A. Lwoff, made extensive research on the physiology of fever, and he concluded that:

"High temperature during infection helps combat the growth of virus. Therefore, fever should not be brought down with drugs."

Artificially induced fever, used extensively by ancient doctors, has been revived in modern practice by Maria Schlenz of Germany. The famous Schlenz-bath, which she originated, is now used extensively in many biological clinics in Europe. Artificially raised fever is the cornerstone in the therapeutic program of two of the most famous cancer clinics in the world — Dr. Issels' Ringberg Clinic, and Dr. Zabel's Berchtesgaten Clinic, in Germany. More and more progressive doctors are beginning to understand the true nature of fever and are applying it for healing and preventing disease.

How fever "works"

Your body is equipped with the most intricate and effective protective and healing system. When you subject yourself to various stresses of life, or when your body is attacked by hostile organisms, your defensive system initiates various protective measures to meet the demands of stress. A complex glandular system — particularly the lymphatic glands, tonsils, and endocrine glands — forms a defensive line against hostile invaders, poisons, or other stress factors which pose a threat to your health or your life. If this first line of defense is broken, your body initiates more drastic measures for correcting the conditions that threaten your health. Fever is one of these defensive and healing measures. The high temperature speeds up metabolism, inhibits the growth of the invading virus or bacteria, and literally burns the enemy with heat. This is not wishful thinking, but a solidly established scientific fact, proven by Dr. A. Lwoff in many experiments. Fever is an effective protective and healing measure, not only against colds, simple infections, and muscular pains, but also such serious ailments as polio, cancer, rheumatic diseases, skin disorders, and insomnia.

How Finns use fever to stay healthy and young

While modern medical science is in the process of discovering the therapeutic benefits of fever, Finnish people have been using artificially created fever for centuries. After discovering instinctively the invigorating, health-promoting, and rejuvenating effect of heat on their bodies, Finns have built steam-bath houses — saunas — and have made sauna-bathing a national tradition unparalleled in history. In fact, Finland, this little, cold Northern country with the rugged, honest, and brave people, is known around the world mainly for three reasons: (1) It is the only country that has paid all of its debts to the United States; (2) It is the only country that won its war with Russia and retained independence (1939-40); and (3) It is the originator of the now famous sauna, the popularity of which is spreading world-wide.

Sauna, the Finnish steambath, is an historic tradition in Finland. For over a thousand years, the sauna has been an important part of Finnish life and Finnish culture — cherished by every Finnish man, woman, and child. The sauna is credited with being a most important reason for the rugged vitality and endurance — the *sisu* — of the Finnish people; also for their exceptional health and low incidence of such degenerative diseases as cancer and arthritis.

In a country of less than 5 million people, there are an estimated 700,000 steam bath facilities — one sauna for every 7 people! Most Finnish saunas are in buildings specially constructed for this purpose. Every farm has its own sauna, normally built on the shore of a lake or river. Most family dwellings in the city have a sauna built on the lot, usually in the back yard. In most apartment buildings, a special sauna room is constructed in the basement. All cities and towns have a large number of public saunas where those few Finns who do not have their own private saunas go at least once or twice a week.

The traditional Finnish sauna is a so-called smoke sauna. It is a timber structure, about 12 by 18 feet, divided into two chambers — the dressing room, and the steam room. The dressing room has several benches to rest on while cooling down after the bath. The steam room has a large oven built from field stones, which are heated by a wood fire. There is no smoke chimney — smoke fills the room while the sauna is being heated up. There is a large iron cauldron built into the oven for hot water. A barrel of cold water is also in the bathing room. There is a window, and a ventilation shutter. Stair-type benches of various heights are built on one side of the room. The sauna is ready for use when the rocks in the oven are hot. Then the fire is put out, the room is well ventilated to remove the rest of the smoke, and the sauna is ready. Of course, the more modern types of Finnish sauna are now built so that the smoke does not enter the room at all, although rocks are always used. In some newer models, the rocks are heated by electric heat.

In Finland, the whole family normally takes a bath together. Sometimes, especially in large families with servants and guests, all the men go together first, then all the women join in a group bath. The sauna is always taken on Saturday evenings, sometimes also in the middle of the week.

The Finnish sauna starts with *löyly*, which is the Finnish word for steam. Water is thrown over the hot rocks, hot steam fills the room and raises the temperature. The bather can sit on the desired level of the stair-like benches, depending on the temperature he perfers — the higher the bench, the higher the temperature. The usual temperature for a Finnish sauna is about 212 degrees F, sometimes even higher. However, for the uninitiated, I would not advise temperatures higher than 180-190 degrees F.

In order to further increase the effect of heat and to stimulate sweating and raise the body's temperature, the Finns use birch brooms — *vihta*. Fresh birch branches with leaves are tied together to form a short broom. They are used fresh in summer, or dried in winter. The dried broom is dipped in warm water and it immediately regains the same shape as the fresh one. Bathers hit themselves all over with these birch brooms. It may seem odd and eccentric to the uninitiated, but you have to try it yourself to appreciate the fantastic delight and unbelievable pleasure that sauna with a birch broom can give!

Following the sauna with hot *löyly*, bathers wash themselves with warm water and soap, and then take a long, relaxing rest on the benches in the dressing room, allowing their wide-open pores to close slowly, perspiration to cease, and the body to return slowly to normal temperature.

Since saunas are becoming more and more popular in the United States, and since there is so much misunderstanding and misinformation regarding the correct way to build and use the sauna, I wish to emphasize these two points:

1. The Finnish sauna is never a *dry* sauna. The heat in the authentic Finnish sauna is always created by throwing water over the hot rocks — thus, it is a moist, steam heat.

2. Finns do not end their saunas by cooling themselves rapidly with a cold shower, as is often advised in the United States. Even when Finns, while taking a sauna, swim in the lake or river, or roll in the soft snow during the winter, they always go back to the hot sauna for a second session, and then finish the whole ceremony by taking a long rest on the dressing room bench and letting the body return *slowly* to normal temperature. This is important, as the healing and rejuvenating effects of the sauna are largely due to the raised body temperature, and to cool it down suddenly with a cold shower would be to interrupt a beneficial process and could possibly cause harm.

Why Sauna heals and rejuvenates.

The therapeutic and rejuvenative property of sauna is attributed to the following facts:

- Overheating with *löyly* stimulates and speeds up the metabolic processes and inhibits the growth of pathogenic bacteria or virus.
- The vital organs and glands, including endocrine and sex glands, are stimulated to increased activity.
- The body's own healing activity and restorative capacity are accelerated and increased. The healing of many chronic and acute conditions, such as colds, infections, rheumatic diseases, and cancer is accelerated by the body's own curative forces.
- The body is thoroughly cleansed and rejuvenated inside and outside. Sauna brings about profuse sweating. Many toxins, accumulated in the system as a result of metabolic wastes and sluggish elimination, are thrown out of the body with perspiration. The skin is our largest eliminative organ — 30% of all body wastes are normally eliminated by way of perspiration. The chemical analysis of sweat shows that it contains almost the same constituents as urine (skin is appropriately called our "third kidney"). The sauna increases the eliminative, detoxifying, and cleansing capacity of the skin by the stimulating action on the sweat glands.

It is easy to see why Finnish people are known for their rugged health, stamina, and youthful vigor.

How you can use fever for health and rejuvenation.

If you are fortunate enough to have your own sauna, or have access to one, take a sauna once or twice a week. Follow the Finnish method, and *do not cool yourself with a cold shower immediately after the sauna.* Wrap yourself in a large bath towel to preserve the body heat, and let your body cool down slowly by resting for half an hour or longer.

If you do not have access to a sauna, you can benefit from overheating therapy by taking a Schlenz-bath regularly, or by taking an improvised do-it-yourself sauna in your bed. Here's how you do it.

SCHLENZ-BATH

Fill your bath tub with warm water, about 98 degrees F. If you don't have a large enough tub to enable you to cover your whole body with water, plug the emergency outlet with a piece of cloth or paper so that the water level can be raised (but be careful not to flood your house!). Stay *under* the water as completely as possible, leaving only the face out for breathing. Let hot water run slowly from the faucet so that the temperature of the water will be gradually raised to 102 or 103 degrees F., possibly even higher. After about half an hour, your body temperature will match the temperature of the water, if you are totally immersed. Then dry yourself, wrap with a large, dry bath towel, and go to bed, covered with a warm blanket. Stay in bed and continue sweating for as long as possible — maybe an hour or more — until your body temperature gradually returns to normal.

Note: 1. Do not eat for at least two hours before bath.
2. Those who suffer from any kind of illness, but particularly heart disease, should ask their doctor about the advisability of using hot baths, and should abide by his expert advise.

DO-IT-YOURSELF SAUNA

Wrap yourself in a large, heavy bath towel. Put a plastic or rubber sheet on your bed to protect it from damage from perspiration. Take two or three hot water bottles (or electric heating pads) and lay on the rubber sheet. Cover yourself with an electric blanket turned on high, leaving just a crack for breathing. Use several heavy blankets if necessary. Remain until profuse sweating occurs — half an hour or more. Then dry yourself and rest in bed again for a while until the body is slowly cooled down.

Finally, a piece of good advice: physical activity to the point of heavy perspiration, is almost as beneficial, if not more so, than the overheating bath. Physical exertion may actually raise body temperature several degrees. A combination of regular heavy exercise, such as running, jogging, or active games, resulting in profuse perspiration, can substitute for a Finnish sauna.

FINNISH HEALTH AND REJUVENATION
SECRET NUMBER TWO – RYE

My world-wide studies show that all people known for their excellent health always use some kind of grain as a staple in their diet. In Russia, it is buckwheat and millet. In Mexico, it is corn and beans. In China, it is rice and millet. In the Middle East, it is sesame seeds. In East Europe, it is barley. In Scotland, it is oats. Grains, seeds, and nuts are the most important and most potent foods for man's health. Their nutritional value is unsurpassed by any other food. Eaten mostly raw and sprouted, but also cooked, they contain all the important nutrients essential for human growth, maintenance of health, and prevention of disease in the most perfect combination and balance. In addition, they contain the secret of life itself – *the germ* – the reproductive power that assures the perpetuation of the species. This reproductive power is of extreme importance for the life of man, his health, and his own reproductive capacity.

All seeds and grains are useful and beneficial, but some grains are more so than others. Millet and buckwheat contain complete proteins of high quality, which most other grains do not contain. Rye, wheat, rice and corn do not contain all the essential amino acids which form high quality proteins. Furthermore, many vital nutrients in grains, such as minerals, and particularly the trace minerals manganese, iron, copper, molybdenum, and zinc, are not well utilized by the body as they are "locked in" by phytin, which the human digestive system is unable to break down.

Rye has been a staple in the Finnish diet for centuries, mostly in the form of rye bread. But Finns eat mostly *sour rye bread*, which is one of the secrets of their exceptional health. According to Dr. Johannes Kuhl (see the next chapter), the famous German expert on soured (lactic acid) foods, the fermentation of grains makes many nutrients more easily available for assimilation in the intestinal tract. During the natural souring process in making a sour-dough bread, the phytin is broken down and valuable minerals and trace elements are released. Also, during the fermentation, due to the enzymatic action on the grain, valuable lactic acid develops – an extremely beneficial health-promoting and disease-preventing factor, as demonstrated by Dr. Kuhl and others in actual studies.

Sour rye bread is also extremely beneficial for the health of the digestive and eliminative organs. Being a "predigested" food, it is easily digested and utilized even by weak organs. It is also an *anti-constipation food* – while most other grains are just the opposite! And, as you remember from the previous chapter, chronic constipation is one of the prime causes of most degenerative diseases, as well as of premature aging. Here's how to make

SOURDOUGH RYE BREAD

8 cups freshly ground whole rye flour
3 cups warm water
½ cup sourdough culture

Mix seven cups of flour with water and sourdough culture. Cover and let stand in a warm place overnight – between 12 and 18 hours. Add remaining flour and mix well. Place in greased pans. Let rise for approximately half hour. Bake at 350 degrees one hour, or more if needed. Always save a half cup of dough as a culture for the next baking. Keep culture in a tightly closed jar in your refrigerator. For the initial baking it will be necessary to obtain a sourdough culture from a commercial bakery. This recipe makes two two-pound loaves.

3

Rejuvenation Secrets from GERMANY

Germans are perhaps more health conscious than any other people I know. They have, for example, the thousands-of-years-long tradition of *bads* — health spas, mineral baths and hot springs, where they go for a *cure*. There are several hundreds of famous *bads* in Germany, where an estimated 3 million people go each year to improve their health, cure disease, and/or prevent sickness. The private industries and insurance companies in Germany spent an estimated 20 million dollars setting up so-called health rebuilding centers, where executives and workers are sent periodically to have their health rebuilt, their heart conditions corrected, and where they are instructed to follow a special regimen and a diet upon their return home, in order to prevent recurrance.

Germany, where modern medical science was born, also leads the world in regard to the "medical science of the future" — biological medicine. Over 3,000 German medical doctors are members of the Society of Biological Doctors, who do not use drugs, but adhere to the naturopathic methods of natural healing. There are over 300 biological clinics in Germany run by these doctors, where millions of people are treated yearly.* Many of the most successful biological approaches and methods of treatment have originated in these clinics. I will introduce you to some of these treatments.

---

* A full page of addresses of some of these clinics, also some biological clinics in Sweden and Switzerland, is printed in my book, "There Is a Cure for Arthritis", Parker Publishing Co., West Nyack, N.Y., 1968. Available at most health food stores and book stores.

FERMENTED FOODS

I don't know if the Germans originated sauerkraut, but it has been an essential part of the German diet for centuries. Germans also use a lot of other fermented foods such as black sour bread, sour pickles, and soured or pickled vegetables, such as green and red peppers, beets, carrots, etc.

Fermented foods are used in Germany and many East-European countries not only as a food, but also as a medicine. Miraculous cures of arthritis, scurvy, ulcers, colds, digestive disorders, even cancer, have been attributed to the regular use of fermented foods. People have been eating these foods for centuries without knowing why they had such a curative effect.

Now, German cancer researcher, Dr. Johannes Kuhl, M.D., gives us a scientific explanation as to why fermented foods not only can build health and prevent disease, but also cure disease. "Natural lactic acid and fermentive enzymes, which are produced during the fermentation process, have a beneficial effect on metabolism and a curative effect on disease." says Dr. Kuhl.

Lactic acid destroys harmful bacteria in the intestines and contributes to the better digestion and assimilation of nutrients. Fermented foods can be considered to be predigested foods — very easily digested and assimilated even by persons with weak digestive organs. Fermented foods improve intestinal hygiene and provide a proper nourishment for the body's own vitamin production within the intestines. They are also excellent preventative foods against constipation.

You can see now why fermented foods, such as sauerkraut, pickled vegetables, sour black bread and soured milks were always regarded by those who use them regularly as health-building and rejuvenating foods.

Here are a few tips regarding fermented foods:

Do not use commercial sauerkraut or sour pickles from your regular supermarket. They are always prepared with vinegars (not to mention several toxic chemicals and preservatives) and can not be considered to be natural lactic acid foods. In fact, they do not contain natural lactic acid.

Make your own fermented foods. Here are some recipes

and instructions for homemade sauerkraut, homemade sour pickles, pickled vegetables and soured milks.

HOMEMADE SOURED MILK

Use only unpasteurized, raw milk. Place a bottle of milk in a pan filled with warm water and warm it to about body temperature. Fill a cup or a deep plate, stir in a tablespoon of yogurt, cover with a paper towel (for dust) and keep in a warm place – for example, near the stove, radiator, or wherever there is a constant warm temperature. The milk will coagulate in approximately 24 hours.

Use one or two spoonfuls of soured milk as a culture for your next batch (use yogurt or commercial buttermilk only as a starting culture for the first batch).

HOMEMADE KEFIR

To make your own kefir, you will need kefir grains. There is a mail order company, R. J. Biological Laboratory, 35 Park Ave., Blue Point, Long Island, New York, which sells kefir grains by mail directly to customers. The kefir grains will last indefinitely – there is never any need to reorder. Merely follow the instructions which will come with each order.

Place 1 tbsp. of kefir grains in a glass of milk, stir and allow to stand at room temperature overnight. When the milk coagulates, it is ready for eating. Kefir is a true "elixir of youth" used by centenarians in Bulgaria, Russia, and Caucasus as a part of their daily diet.

HOMEMADE YOGURT

Take a bottle of skim milk and heat it almost to boiling. Let stand to cool down to body temperature. Add two to three tablespoons of yogurt, which can be bought in a grocery store or health shop. Stir well. Pour into a wide-mouthed thermos bottle. Cover and let stand overnight. In five to eight hours, it will be solid and ready to serve. If you do not have a thermos jar, use an ordinary glass jar and place it in a pan of warm water over an electric burner switched on "warm" for four to five hours, then switch off until milk is solid.

Use two to three spoonfuls of your fresh homemade yogurt as a culture for the next batch.

HOMEMADE SAUERKRAUT

Use a small wooden barrel, or a large earthernware pot. Possibly a large stainless steel pail or a glass jar could be used, but under no circumstances use an aluminum utensil.

Cut white cabbage heads into narrow strips with a large knife or grater, and place in a barrel. When the layer of cabbage is about four to six inches deep, sprinkle a few juniper berries, cummin seeds, and/or black currant leaves on top – use your favorite or whatever you have available. A few strips of carrots, green peppers, and onions can also be used. Add a little sea salt – not more than two ounces for each 25 pounds of cabbage. Then add another layer of grated cabbage and spices until the container is filled. Each layer should be pressed and stamped very hard with your fists or a piece of wood so that there will be no air left and the cabbage will be saturated with its own juice.

When the container is full, cover cabbage with a clean linen canvas or cheese cloth, place a wooden or slate board over it, and on the top, place a clean heavy stone. Let stand for two to three weeks in a warm place, not below 70 degrees F. Now and then remove the foam and the possible mildew from the top, from the stone, and from the barrel edges. The linen canvas, board, and stone, should be occasionally removed, washed well with warm water and then cold water, and replaced. After about three weeks, the sauerkraut is ready for eating. It can be left in the barrel, which should now be stored in a cool place, or put in glass jars and kept in the refrigerator.

Sauerkraut is best eaten *raw* – both from the standpoint of taste and for its health-giving value. Drink sauerkraut juice, too. It is an extremely beneficial and wonderfully nutritious drink.

HOMEMADE PICKLED VEGETABLES

Use the same method as described above for homemade sauerkraut to make health-giving lactic acid vegetables. Beets, carrots, green and red peppers, beet tops, swiss chard, and celery are particularly adapted for pickling.

HOMEMADE SOUR PICKLES

Use only small, fresh, hard cucumbers. Place them in cold water overnight, then dry them well.

Place cucumbers in a wooden barrel, or a large earthenware or glass jar. Place a few leaves of black currants, cherries, mustard seeds, and plenty of dill branches in with the cucumbers.

Boil a sufficient amount of salt water, using about four ounces of sea salt for five quarts of water. Let water cool down, then pour it over the cucumbers. Cover with linen canvas or cheese cloth, place a wooden board over it, and on top a clean heavy stone. There should be enough salt water to cover the board. Keep the container in a warm place for about one week, then move to a cooler place. Pickles are ready for eating in about three to four weeks. Every second week or so, remove the stone and the covers and wash them well, first in warm water, then in cold water; then replace them. Keep the top of the water clean of foam and mildew. When pickles are ready for eating, they can be placed in glass jars and kept in the refrigerator.

You can now also buy many lactic acid vegetables and juices in cans or bottles, imported from Germany and Switzerland – these can be found in most health food stores.

Not only Germans, but also most other people known for their exceptionally good health and long life use lots of fermented foods in their diet – Hunzas, Russians, Bulgarians, Japanese, even North American Indians. If you wish to enjoy good health, prevent disease, and live long, perhaps you can follow their example and include some fermented foods in your rejuvenation diet.

MINERAL WATERS

As I said previously, Germany is famous for its *bads* – mineral bathing and drinking spas where over three million people go each year to heal and rejuvenate themselves.

The water cure is an old tradition in Germany. Cities have

been built around mineral-rich springs. Most mineral-spring spas are operated by the city or municipal governments and are directed by licensed medical doctors. In Germany, doctors don't frown on the mineral spas as quackery, as American doctors do. On the contrary, most patients who frequent bathing places for a water cure, are sent there by their doctors.

I have visited many *bads* in Germany, and interviewed many doctors who operate them, as well as many patients who take the water cure. All were enthusiastic regarding the benefits of drinking mineral waters and taking mineral baths. High blood pressure, arthritis, female disorders, cardio-vascular diseases, skin disorders, nervous disorders, allergies, diseases of old age and senility — this is just a partial list of diseases improved or cured in these water spas.

How mineral waters heal and rejuvenate

There is a new branch of medical science that many researchers in Germany are probing with an intensified inquiry. It is called *Balnealogy* — the medical science of curing and preventing sickness by bathing.

A doctor in one of the most famous bathing places in Germany, Bad Pyrmont, told me:

"The modern inquiry into balnealogy and the medicinal value of mineral waters is recent and as yet incomplete. But what is already known indicates that mineral waters do indeed have curative powers. And they should, inasmuch as disordered mineral metabolism and biochemical derangement are at the root of many diseases. But what is even more important is the fact that these waters here in Bad Pyrmont have been used for healing purposes for almost two thousand years; and millions of sick people have benefited by them — patients and doctors see examples of it every day!"

For many years, it was believed that our bodies can only use *organic* minerals, and that *inorganic* minerals, such as those present in mineral waters, can not be utilized by the body, and can even be harmful. Now, scientists have reversed their opinions completely. Several studies from around the world show that, actually, inorganic minerals are not only well utilized, but that they are of extreme importance in the maintenance of health.

Drs. Korenyi, Harkavy, and Whittier reported on the experiments they conducted with 35 patients with high cholserol levels at the Creedmore State Hospital in New York. These patients, whose serum cholesterol levels were above 240 mg. %, did not receive any other type of treatment known to have any effect on serum cholesterol, except 30½ fluid ounces of mineral water daily in three divided doses. The treatment continued for 30 days. At the end of two weeks, the average decrease of serum cholesterol was 9.9 mg. %. At the conclusion of the study, the average decrease was 23.8 mg. %.

A Hungarian doctor, O. Schulhof, M. D., made a study of the spa therapies and reported that "Besides the psychological effects produced by the changed environment and the complex effect of various treatments, we still attribute importance to the specific effect of the mineral water." Dr. Schulhof said that it has been demonstrated that mineral water is actually absorbed through the skin during bathing. Mineral waters have been shown to have a beneficial effect on the connective tissues as well as on the immunological and healing powers of the body.

I have a first hand experience with the value of mineral waters. During several years, I directed a biological clinic at a hot mineral spring spa in Mexico. We used mineral waters for bathing as well as for drinking. We have seen many striking examples of recovery from a multitude of acute and chronic conditions. I can agree with Dr. Schulhof, that besides the complex effect of fasting, diet, and other therapies, I still attribute the remarkable results, at least in part, to the specific effect of mineral water.

Extensive studies in Europe and the United States showed that wherever people drink hard water (naturally heavily mineralized water) they have less heart disease, less tooth decay, less hardening of the arteries, and less diabetes than those who live in areas where soft water is used. Striking evidence comes from Monroe Country, Florida, where the water supply was suddenly changed from rain water, with a hardness of .5 parts per million, to deep well water with a hardness 400 times greater. The death rate from heart disease and blood vessel diseases dropped from the 500 -700 range to the 200-300 level within four years after the increase in water hardness *(Journal of American Dietetic Association,* Vol. 62., June 1973., p. 631).

I have stressed the danger of drinking soft, and especially distilled water in several of my books. *"Are You Confused?"* contains a chapter, 'The Water Controversies', where I presented ample evidence that prolonged use of distilled water can be extremely harmful, and that minerals in hard water should form an essential part of our mineral nutrition. In spite of this, many people, still confused and brainwashed by some books and pamphlets on the subject, continue to drink distilled water, thereby damaging their health and shortening their lives.

Sea water — mineral gold mine

Those who live close to the ocean can benefit from the rejuvenating and health-restoring effect of sea water minerals by frequent bathing in salt water, and also by drinking it.

Sea water is extremely rich in beneficial minerals. One or two tablespoons of pure sea water a day can be used internally as a mineral supplement. Some health food stores now sell purified sea water.

Minerals from the sea are also absorbed through the skin and through the inhaled mineral-rich air by the seashore. Make every effort to spend your holiday by the sea. In addition to providing the usual benefits of cold water bathing, salt water and salt air will recharge your system with health-restoring and rejuvenating minerals.

JUICE FASTING

Perhaps the greatest contribution the Germans have given to the art and science of maintaining good health and enjoying long life, is the development of the newest and most effective form of fasting — JUICE FASTING.

Fasting is not a German discovery, of course. It has been practiced throughout medical history, even before the advent of organized medicine. In fact, fasting is the oldest therapeutic method known to man. But, until just a few decades ago, the only form of fasting employed by practitioners was a traditional, classic form of fasting — a pure water fast, the abstinence from all foods and drinks with the exception of pure water. Most American practitioners and health clinics still employ this antiquated form of fasting.

In Europe, and particularly in Germany, a few pioneers of biological medicine began experimenting with a different form of fasting. The result was that now the traditional water fast is never employed in any of the spas and clinics in Europe. It is replaced with the juice fast, or Rohsäfte-Kur, which all the leading fasting authorities in Germany have found to be superior to water fasting — more effective in healing disease and bringing about a more thorough cleansing and rejuvenation of the tissues.*

The scientific justification of the superiority of juice fasting is based on the following physiological facts:

1. The main cause of disease and aging are to be found in the derangement of normal processes of cell metabolism and cell regeneration. The accumulation of toxins and metabolic waste products interferes with the nourishment of the cells and slows down cell regeneration and new cell building. When the normal metabolic processes become deranged, due to nutritional deficiencies, sluggish digestion and elimination, sedentary life, and overeating, and the process of cell nourishment, replacement and rebuilding slows down, your body starts to grow old, its resistance to disease will diminish, and various ills will start to appear. Keep in mind that only about half of your cells are in the peak of development, vitality and working condition. One fourth are usually in the process of development and growth, and the other fourth in the process of breaking down or dying. The healthy vital life processes and perpetual youth are maintained when there is perfect balance in this process of cell breakdown and replacement. If the cells are breaking down and dying at a faster rate than the new cells are built, the process of aging will begin to set in. Also, it is of vital

---

* One of the originators of juice fasting is Dr. Eugene Heun, M. D., Ph.D. Other leading juice fast specialists in Germany are Dr. Otto Buchinger, Jr. and Dr. Werner Zabel.

importance that the aging and dying cells are decomposed and eliminated as soon as possible. Quick and effective elimination of dead cells stimulates the building and growth of new cells.

Here is where juice fasting comes in as the most effective way to restore your health and rejuvenate your body. During a juice fast, the process of elimination of the dead and dying cells is speeded up, and the building of new cells is accelerated and stimulated.

2. During a juice fast, the eliminative and cleansing capacity of the eliminative organs — lungs, liver, kidneys, bowels, and skin — is greatly increased and masses of accumulated metabolic wastes and toxins are quickly expelled.

3. Juice fasting exerts a normalizing, stabilizing and re-juvenating effect on all the vital physiological, nervous and mental functions. The nervous system is rejuvenated; mental powers are improved; glandular chemistry and hormonal secretions are stimulated.

4. Vitamin deficiencies and mineral imbalance in the tissues is one of the main causes of diminished oxygenation of cells, which leads to disease and premature aging of cells. Raw juices are rich in vitamins, enzymes, and minerals and trace elements. These are easily assimilated directly into the blood-stream and help to restore biochemical and mineral balance in the tissues and cells, and, thus, help to speed recovery and rejuvenate the tissues.

5. Overacidity in the tissues is one of the main causes of disease. Especially during fasting, blood and tissues contain large amounts of acids as a result of autolysis, or self-digestion. Raw juices provide an alkaline surplus, which is extremely important for the proper acid-alkaline balance.

6. According to Dr. Ralph Bircher, raw juices contain an as yet unidentified factor which stimulates what he calls a "micro-electric tension" in the body, and is responsible for the cells' ability to absorb nutrients from the blood stream and effectively excrete metabolic wastes.

Thus, raw juices are of particular importance when you fast for the regeneration and rejuvenation of your body. Juice fasting will help to break down and dispose of old, dying cells, revitalize the active cells, and accelerate the building of young vital cells.

Here's what Dr. Ragnar Berg, perhaps the world's greatest authority on nutrition and biochemistry, said about the superiority of juice fasting over water fasting:

"During fasting, the body burns up and excretes huge amounts of accumulated wastes. We can help this cleansing process by drinking alkaline juices instead of water while fasting. I have supervised many fasts, and made extensive tests of fasting patients, and I am convinced that drinking alkaline-forming fruit and vegetable juices instead of water during fasting will increase the healing effect of fasting. The elimination of uric acid and other inorganic acids will be accelerated. And sugars in juices will strengthen the heart. Juice fasting is, therefore, the best form of fasting."

The foremost fasting authority in the world, Dr. Otto H. F. Buchinger, Jr., M. D., has directed and supervised over 80,000 fasts in his clinic (more than any other doctor in the world). He told me that he employs only juice fasting, because, in his experience, "fasting on fresh raw juices of fruits and vegetables, plus vegetable broths and herb teas, results in much faster recovery from disease and more effective cleansing and rejuvenation of the tissues than does the traditional water fast."

I have studied various methods of fasting for several decades in several countries. Among my teachers in biological medicine and fasting I am proud to count Are Waerland, Ragnar Berg, Werner Zabel, and Otto Buchinger, Jr. — all leading fasting authorities. I have also had personal experience with directing and supervising the fasting of hundreds of patients, and observing the results of various fasting methods on specific conditons. I can testify that juice fasting is, indeed, superior to water fasting. It is the best, safest, and most effective healing method I know. Juice fasting not only accomplishes a physiological rejuvenation and revitalization of your body, but also has a profound effect on your mind and mental facilities. It stimulates and sharpens mental and aesthetic perception and increases your spiritual awareness.

Juice fasting — this modern, scientific health-restoring and rejuvenating miracle — will recharge, renew, and rejuvenate your whole personality — physically, sexually, mentally, and spiritually.

(For a complete description of the philosophy and mechanics of juice fasting, and for detailed instructions for do-it-yourself fast, see my book, *How to Keep Slim, Healthy and Young with Juice Fasting.*, available at all leading health food stores, or from HEALTH PLUS, Publishers, P. O. Box 22001, Phoenix, Arizona 85028).

4

REJUVENATION SECRETS
FROM
BULGARIA

As I mentioned in the first chapter. Ilja Metchnikoff, the famous Russian scientist, revolutionized medical thinking on aging when he published his famous theory on the prolongation of life by preventing autotoxemia due to colonic putrefaction and the development of toxins in the colon.

Metchnikoff made studies of the Bulgarian eating habits, and he become convinced that their exceptional longevity is the result of their special diet. It is well known that Bulgarians consume more soured milk in the form of yogurt and kefir than do people of any other nation. Metchnikoff claimed that the generous and continuous use of soured milk products such as yogurt, kefir, acidophilus milk, etc., helps to prevent putrefaction in the colon and the consequent autotoxemia or self-poisoning – thus, improving health and prolonging life.

Bulgarians seem to be living proof of Dr. Metchnikoff's theory. They are healthy and tall people – the tallest people in Europe. They also live longer than most other people on earth. They have more centenarians – people who live to be 100 or more – than any other civilized nation. According to statistics they have 1,600 centenarians for every one million people, as compared to only seven persons 100 years or older per million in the United States.

Bulgarians are known to retain the characteristics of youth to an advanced age. The virility of their "old" men is legendary.

There is extensive literature to support yogurt as a youthifying food. We must keep in mind, however, that the yogurt consumed by most Bulgarian centenarians is not made from cow's milk, but from sheep's or goat's milk. It is well known that the health-building and youth-preserving qualities of sheep's and goat's milk are superior to those of cow's milk. The protein and mineral composition of goat's or sheep's milk is closer to that of human milk than is cow's milk. Goat's milk contains anti-cancer and anti-arthritis factors, which may account in part for its life prolonging property.

Yogurt is not the only Bulgarian secret for a long, healthy life. My study of Bulgarian centenarians and their living and eating habits revealed that they adhere to many other health-building and rejuvenating living habits:

- Most of them are predominantly lacto-vegetarians. That is, their diet consists mostly of locally-grown and freshly stone ground whole grains (especially barley), and fresh vegetables and fruits from their own gardens. They eat very little meat. Only about 3 or 4 percent of all centenarians eat meat regularly.
- Most Bulgarian centenarians are bee keepers and use lots of honey in their diet.
- They consume lots of fermented foods — especially sauerkraut. As you have seen in the previous chapter, fermented foods help to prevent and cure many diseases, and, thus, prolong life.
- Almost all of them eat sunflower seeds as an essential part of their diet.
- They live "close to nature" following nature's rhythm in working, eating, and sleeping; they are usually poor to the extent that they can not afford to overeat; they are engaged in hard physical work; they are friendly, contented, and have no great ambitions or jealousy.

Here we have it: a blueprint for a happy, healthy, and long life. No fancy secrets, tricky diets or drugs — just simple common sense natural foods and wholesome stress-free country living. But don't be deceived by its apparent simplicity: the factors mentioned — a lacto-vegetarian diet, yogurt, honey, sunflower seeds, fermented foods, and moderate eating — all are sceintifically proven to be potent factors in preventing premature aging and prolonging life.

5

REJUVENATION SECRETS
FROM
RUSSIA

Russians are far ahead of other countries in research on longevity. While in the United States, preoccupation with rejuvenation or attempts to prolong one's life are considered by most scientists to be an oddity at best, if not innane health-faddist notions, in the USSR, the prolongation of life is a legitimate science. There are several research institutes on longevity financed by the government. Extensive research has been going on at these research centers for decades. Russian medical scientists consider the prevention of disease and prolongation of life as their ultimate goals. Well-known Russian physiologist, Tarkhanov, wrote:

"The time will come when it will be a disgrace for a man to die less than 100 years old."

One of the Soviet scientists engaged in research on longevity is Olga Lepeshinskaya. In her book, *LIFE, AGE AND LONGE-VITY*, she states that the normal life span of human beings should not be less than *150 years*, if they would observe the elementary laws of health. Everyone who feels old before he reaches 100, she says, is suffering from premature old age. She claims that premature aging, like other diseases, can be prevented. It can also be successfully treated after it appears. How? Here's her recipe:

- Sound, simple, natural nutrition.
- Plenty of physical work, recreation, and rest.
- Cheerful, optimistic outlook on life.

We must agree that this simple program will "work" for anyone who will conscientiously apply it in his life.

Of the many rejuvenation secrets that the Russians have discovered, I will bring to you a few of the more important ones. I have made extensive travels and studies in Russia, and I can assure you that the Russians are indeed superior to us as far as health and longevity is concerned. They are known for their endurance and stamina. They have seven times more centenarians per million than the United States. Their mortality rate is 7.3 per thousand as compared to 9.4 per thousand in the United States. The life expectancy of the Russian male is 70.1 — the American male's is only 66.7 years. In Abkhazia, the Russian province in Caucasus where most centenarians live, the average life expectancy for both men and women is over 100 years!

POLLEN-RICH HONEY

The discovery of pollen-rich honey as a life prolonger was made in the course of research in one of the Longevity Institutes in Russia. The famed Russian scientist, biologist, and experimental botanist, Dr. Nicolai Tsitsin, was engaged in research on longevity. The aim of his inquiry was to find ways of prolonging human life.

"We decided to send letters to 200 people claiming to be over 100 years old with the request to answer the following three questions: what was their age; how had they earned their living most of their lives; and what had been their principle food."

Dr. Tsitsin received 150 replies to his 200 letters.

"We made a very interesting discovery. The answers showed that a large number of them were bee keepers. And *all of them*, without exception, said that their principle food had always been honey!"

But as sensational as this discovery was, this was not all!

"We found, continued Dr. Tsitsin, "that in each case, it wasn't really honey these people ate, but the waste matter in the bottom of the honey containers. Because most bee keepers were poor, they sold all of the pure honey on the market, keeping only the 'dirty residue' for themselves."

After a series of laboratory tests, Dr. Tsitsin discovered that the "dirty residue" of the honey was not a dirt at all, but almost pure pollen, which falls off the bees' legs while they deposit their honey. Thus, Tsitsin discovered one of the most important rejuvenation secrets of Russian centenarians — pollen-rich, natural, unfiltered, and unprocessed honey!

Of course, the fact that honey and pollen are age-retarding and rejuvenating foods isn't really a Russian discovery; they have been considered such since time immemorial. Cave paintings from the Neolithic age show illustrations of honey-combs being gathered for food. Honey has been found in 3,000 year old Egyptian pyramids. Pythagoras, the great Greek scientist, 600 B.C., recommended honey for health and long life. Many other Greek philosophers claimed that pollen held the secret of eternal youth. The original Olympic athletes used unstrained pollen-rich honey for extra energy and vitality. Throughout the ages, honey and pollen have been regarded as *ambrosia* — divine foods with age-retarding and rejuvenating properties.

The miraculous rejuvenative property of pollen-rich honey is attributed to the fact that pollen is nature's own propagator of life. It is the male germ cell of the plant kingdom. Pollen, in addition to all known water-soluble vitamins — including B_{12} — and a rich supply of minerals, trace elements, and enzymes, contains *deoxiribosides* and *sterines,* plus *steroid* hormone substances. Pollen also contains a gonadotropic *hormone,* a plant hormone which is similar to the pituitary hormone, *gonadotropin,* which stimulates sex glands.

During the last two decades, much research has been done, mostly in Russia and Sweden, to uncover the medicinal and rejuvenative value of pollen and honey. Both have been found to be miraculous rejuvenators, largely by improving general health, preventing disease, increasing the power of the body's own immunological mechanism, and stimulating and rejuvenating glandular activity.

Until 1952, the only pollen available was bee-gathered pollen. Naturally, the price was astronomical since only very small amounts were available. Then, a Swedish amateur bee keeper, Gösta Carlsson, developed a patented process by which tons of pollen could be collected, without the help of the bees, directly from the field flowers by specially constructed collecting machines. The price of pollen dropped, and it became easily available both for research and consumer purposes.

There is a huge amount of research available on pollen, which shows that it is an effective treatment of such varied disorders as prostate troubles, hemorrhoids, asthma, allergies, disgestive disorders and intestinal putrefaction, chronic bronchitis, multiple sclerosis, gastric ulcers, arthritis, hay fever — and of course, the symptoms of aging.

I have mentioned previously the rejuvenative and health-building property of fermented, lactic-acid foods. French researcher, Dr. Remy Chauvin, reports that pollen seems to have an anti-putrefactive factor similar to that of fermented or lactic acid foods. Pollen destroys harmful bacteria in the intestines and improves assimilation and elimination.

Honey is, of course, an undisputed miracle health-building and age-retarding food. More than any other food it fulfills Hippocrates' requirement for the ideal food: i.e. "Let your food be your medicine — let your medicine be your food."

It has been demonstrated that honey:
- increases calcium retention (so important for staying younger longer);
- increases hemoglobin count and can prevent or cure nutritional anemia (it is rich in iron and copper);
- has a beneficial effect on healing processes in such conditions as arthritis, colds, poor circulation, constipation, liver and kidney disorders, weak heart action, bad complexion, and insomnia;
- is rich in aspartic acid, an important amino acid which is involved in the rejuvenative processes, particularly in the rejuvenation of sex glands.

Now you can understand why pollen-rich honey is such an important health and longevity factor in the diet of all Russian centenarians. Pollen and honey have, indeed, age-retarding, health-building, and rejuvenating properties.

It is difficult to obtain "pollen-contaminated" natural honey in the United States. Most honey sold in supermarkets is filtered, heated, and refined — and free from pollen. Health food stores sell unfiltered honey, which contains some pollen. However, pollen is now available in pure form in powder or tablets at all better health food stores. In your rejuvenation diet, take 1 to 2 tsp. of pollen or 10 tablets every day. And, replace all sugar – including so-called brown sugar – with natural honey.

GARLIC AND ONIONS

At the end of the Second World War, when American troops finally confronted the Russian troops, American soldiers discovered that many Russian soldiers had their pockets filled with onions and garlic, and judging from the odor, they made good use of them. For several years, the Russian Army fought on a near-starvation diet because of a severe food shortage. But two things always seemed to be in good supply: garlic and onions. In addition to buckwheat porridge and black bread, garlic and onions comprised the Russian Army's staple ration.

While traveling in Russia, I enjoyed stopping at the villages and studying the life in the agricultural collectives, their methods of cultivation, preferred crops, etc. In addition to the collectively owned fields, each family was allowed to have a large garden of their own, where they could grow anything they wished for their own use or for sale on the public market. I have found that two vegetables completely dominated these gardens: cabbage (for sauerkraut) and onions!

Russian electrobiologist, Professor Gurwitch, discovered that garlic and onions emit a peculiar type of ultra-violet radiation called mitogenetic radiation. This radiation – the Gurwitch rays – has the property of stimulating cell growth and activity and has a rejuvenating effect on all body functions.

A great amount of scientific research has been done in various countries on the therapeutic properties of garlic and onions. Dr. A. I. Virtanen, Finnish Nobel Prize Winner, discovered 14 *new* beneficial substances in onions. Russian, German, French, English, and American researchers have successfully used garlic to treat such varied conditions as high or low blood pressure, common colds, intestinal worms, cough, asthma, whopping cough, intestinal putrefaction, dysentery, gastrointestinal disorders, gas, tuberculosis, and diabetes. American research has shown that garlic is a powerful agent against tumor formation in cancer. It has also been found to be an effective agent in preventing pneumonia.

Russians discovered that garlic has antibiotic properties. They often refer to garlic as "Russian penicillin." Russian medical clinics and hospitals use garlic extensively — mostly in the form of volatile extracts that are vaporized and inhaled.

I have found in my own practice that the most dramatic therapeutic use of garlic is, perhaps, in the treatment of high blood pressure. Almost without exception, blood pressure can be reduced in two weeks by 30 - 40 mm. by nothing but garlic therapy — including the generous use of raw garlic in the diet. High blood pressure is, of course, one of the causes of heart disease — our greatest killer. The fact that garlic has such a beneficial effect on reducing blood pressure makes it an important life-prolongator. By counteracting intestinal putrefaction and improving assimilation of the essential nutrients from the intestines, garlic and onions improve health and prolong life. Not to mention the fact that garlic and onions also are most delicious foods!

Odor? Well, why not just do like Russians and Italians do: eat and enjoy; let the others worry about our odors!

BUCKWHEAT

During my recent meeting with one of the leading Russian scientists in the field of preventative medicine and longevity, the question came up regarding Russia's low incidence of cardiovascular disease and heart attacks. The Russian scientist said:

"We have a relatively low incidence of high blood pressure and cardiovascular diseases, and we attribute this in part to our regular eating of such foods as garlic and buckwheat. Buckwheat supplies *rutin*, a bioflavonoid, which we have found to have a blood-pressure-reducing property, and a beneficial effect on the circulatory system."

Buckwheat, mostly in the form of a porridge, which they call *kasha,* is really the Russian national food. Wherever I've traveled in Russia, I have seen people eating kasha almost every day of their lives. Kasha is served to all the personnel in the Russian Army several times a week, mostly with sunflower seed oil.

Buckwheat is an extremely nutritious cereal containing complete proteins, vitamins, and minerals — especially manganese and magnesium. It is low in sodium and very rich in potassium. Rutin in buckwheat makes it a very important rejuvenative and age-retarding food, as circulation problems and cardiovascular disorders are at the root of the many aging processes. The proteins in buckwheat are of very high quality, comparable in biological value to proteins in meat and milk, as shown recently by a study of the U. S. Department of Agriculture.

If you wish to try this famous Russian rejuvenative food, here is the recipe and instructions. Buckwheat grains can be bought at most health food stores.

KASHA
(Buckwheat cereal)

1 cup whole buckwheat grains, whole or crushed
2 to 2½ cups of water

Bring water to a boil. Stir the buckwheat into the boiling water and let boil for 2 to 3 minutes. Turn heat to low and simmer for 15 to 20 minutes, stirring occasionally. When all the water is absorbed, remove from the stove and let stand for another 15-30 minutes. Kasha must never be mushy. Serve hot or warm.

Russians eat kasha with sunflower seed oil, butter, or flaxseed oil. My children perfer it with milk and honey. I love it with cold-pressed virgin olive oil. If seasoning is desired, add a little sea salt to the cooking water.

Another way to cook kasha is the way Russians cook it in the country. Mix buckwheat grains in boiling water and place the covered stainless steel or other fire proof pot in an oven heated to 175-200 degrees F. Leave for 3 to 4 hours (for example, make it in the morning and eat it for lunch). Delicious! And it will help keep you younger longer.

OTHER REJUVENATION SECRETS FROM RUSSIA

In addition to pollen-rich honey, garlic and onions, and buckwheat, here are a few other health and longevity secrets from Russia:

1. Russians eat enormous quantities of sunflower seeds and use unrefined cold-pressed sunflower oil. Sunflower oil is rich in vitamin E and essential fatty acides, the deficiency of which is definitely linked with premature aging. Sunflower seeds are also an excellent source of complete protein, B-vitamins, and minerals — especially zinc, which plays an important role in the growth and maturity of the gonads, the male sex glands, and also is vitally linked with the health of the prostate gland. Zinc has been pointed out as an active agent in most so-called virility foods, such as oysters, raw nuts, sea foods, onions, etc.

2. Russians, like Germans, eat lots of fermented lactic acid foods: sourdough bread, sauerkraut, sour pickles, soured milks like kefir, kumis, and plain clabbered milk. All these foods have a rejuvenative effect on the digestive and assimilative tract.

3. Russians eat more natural, unprocessed foods than we do. A very few chemical additives are allowed in food processing, and all artificial colorings and flavorings are totally prohibited.* Cola drinks and chewing gum are not allowed to be sold in Russia.

4. Russians eat very little meat compared to Americans. Their's is a comparatively low-protein diet, and most of their proteins are from vegetable sources. Only 25.5% of their protein intake is acquired from animal sources (in the U. S. - 71%). As I will show you in the chapter on Hunza, over-consumption of animal proteins is one of the surest ways to shorten your life and fall victim to many so-called diseases of civilization, including cancer.

---

* Artificial colorings and flavorings are extremely harmful. Recent studies show that they are the main cause of the growing ranks of overactive, or hyperkinetic, children in this country. American children are fed huge amounts of artificial colorings and flavorings, which they get from soft drinks, processed cereals, and most other foods, including baby foods. Most travelers to Russia have remarked on the well-behaved, well-mannered, contented, and "quiet" Russian children.

6

REJUVENATION SECRETS FROM RUMANIA

On one of my frequent trips to Europe, I met the famous Rumanian doctor, Professor Ana Aslan, M.D., who was very popular in Europe right then. Dr. Aslan discovered the so-called *Gerovital* therapy — the rejuvenation therapy also known as KH-3, procaine, or novacaine therapy. This was in 1968. At 72, Dr. Aslan looked like she could be in the late fifties. Her face was quite free from wrinkles, and even the skin on her arms was perfectly smooth and firm as on a younger person. She was good advertising for her rejuvenation discovery.

About 30 years ago, Dr. Aslan discovered, quite accidentally, that procaine, commonly used as an anesthetic agent, had an age-retarding property. She injected specially designed doses of procaine — which she named H-3 — into patients showing signs of degeneration and premature aging. She observed that stiff, immobile joints became flexible, pain disappeared, and the patients gained new energy and vitality. Since then, Dr. Aslan has improved her original H-3 formula and uses now only a vitamin and hematoporphyrine-enriched formula called *Gerovital,* which she claims has been demonstrated in tests in Italy and the U.S.A. to be superior to pure procaine.

Gerovital has been used in Rumania for over 25 years, and thousands upon thousands of people from Europe and other countries travel to Dr. Aslan's Regeneration Institute in Bucharest to receive Gerovital treatments in modern government-owned clinics under the supervision of dozens ot Aslantrained doctors. Dr. Aslan said that well over 50,000 people have been treated at her Institute.

I have seen many of those who have received treatment at the Bucharest Institute, and also have myself supervised dozens of patients who took KH-3 (the trademark of German-made Gerovital) at our Mexican Spa. I have seen many rather enthusiastic patients who claimed that KH-3 had a revitalizing and rejuvenating effect on them. I have also seen rather dramatic improvements in some patients with chronic degenerative conditions. This is the reason why I decided to share my knowledge of, and my experience with, KH-3 with you, although it is not a natural rejuvenative measure by any means, but a drug. This is not a recommendation or endorsement, just a passing-on of information. Since procaine is not a nutrient, herb, or natural substance, I cannot, being a naturopath, give it my unreserved endorsement. On the other hand, this substance is claimed to be completely harmless and is sold and endorsed for use by the medical governments of many countries, including Switzerland, Holland, Belgium, East and West Germany, Rumania, and Mexico.

Acording to Dr. Aslan, the aging processes start when the body's ability to produce new cells and to replenish the old ones is diminished. Gerovital helps the body to regenerate new cell production, which is the reason for its rejuvenative effect.

KH-3, which is not allowed to be sold in the U.S. at the time of the publication of this book, but which can be bought at most pharmacies in Mexico or European countries, is a special catalyst combination formula which contains hematoporphyrine, an active factor obtained from hemoglobin. It is claimed that hematoporphyrine is an effective synergist of procaine, and that it enhances its regenerative effect. But the catalyst hematoporphyrine by itself affects an improvement in the vital cellular metabolism and glandular functions within the organism in a biological manner.

Those who wish to try KH-3, should take one capsule a day for 3 to 5 months. The treatment can be repeated after a four week pause. Dr. Aslan recommends the taking of KH-3 by all persons over 40 years of age.

Here's what one of my patients wrote to me recently:

"Dear Dr. Airola: You have been in my thoughts as I wanted to write and tell you how grateful I am for all you did for me at the Spa. I can't express adequately the feeling of *joie de vivre* that I had lost, but now have recaptured. Not even when I was a young girl did I feel as well and strong and active as I do now. My day starts at 5:30 a.m., and I am on the go all day — yet I am able to go to evening classes and enjoy them, too! Fasting and the vitamin-mineral program you worked out for me are paying dividends, along with KH-3, dry brush massage, yogurt, rose hips, etc. I am truly beholden to you for giving me back the desire to live and enjoy living — in fact a new lease on life."

Notes: 1. By giving you this information on KH-3 (Gerovital), I do not endorse or recommend it: I only report objectively what I know about it.

2. Please, do not confuse KH-3 (Gerovital), Dr. Ana Aslan's procaine-based product, with H-3, a vitamin product sold in American health food stores. H-3 has *none* of the properties of KH-3, although some irresponsible sellers have been claiming that they are identical.

3. I do not sell KH-3 and am not connected with it, or Dr. Aslan, in any way. Perhaps I should mention in this connection that I do not sell vitamins, food supplements, or other products mentioned in this book, nor do I own or operate any health food stores. I am not in anyway connected with the health food manufacturing or retailing industry, actively or inactively.

7

REJUVENATION SECRETS
FROM
JAPAN

The traditional Japanese diet contains a large percentage of seaweed. In some parts of Japan, as much as one fourth of the daily diet is made up of seaweed in various forms. The Japanese make soups, noodles, casseroles, and other dishes with seaweed.

There are many kinds of edible seaweed. In England and Ireland, the most popular kind is *dulse*, the crisp and tender leaves of which are called "sea lettuce." In Scotland, Norway and Iceland, a seaweed called *porphyra,* which "looks like spinach, and tastes like oysters'', is commonly eaten. In the United States, seaweed called *kelp,* has been extremely popular among health food advocates. The most commonly eaten seaweed in Japan is the same as used in the United States — brown seaweed with large leaves.

The Japanese are among the most vigorous, industrious, and healthy people in the world. Until very recently — before Coca-Cola, McDonalds, and other contributions of "American Culture", moved in, with white bread, sugar, ice cream, soft drinks, milk, meat, etc. — the Japanese enjoyed excellent health and one of the best records of longevity in the East. Their diet was largely vegetarian, with the addition of fish, but almost total absence of meat. One of the staples in their diet was seaweed, or kelp.

Why do I place kelp as one of the most important rejuvenation secrets? Because kelp is a true wonder food of nature, loaded with vital substances not available in any other food.

Kelp is extremely rich in natural iodine, which is essential for the endocrine glands, especially the thyroid. Iodine deficiency can disrupt normal thyroid functions and cause diminished hormone production. Thyroid hormone is largely responsible for your youthful appearance, for your sex appeal, sexual vigor, and libido. Very few foods contain iodine, as most soils, especially in the United States, are deficient in this mineral.

Finnish geologist, Professor V. Auer, warned that man's health and reproductive capacity is in danger because food from depleted soils lacks the minerals and trace elements which are vital for health. For thousands of years, minerals from tilled soils have been washed with the rains and rivers into the sea. These minerals are taken up by the seaweed plants. Seaweed returns to man's diet what soils can no longer supply. The chemical composition of seawater is virtually identical to that of human blood. Thus, seawater contains all the minerals and trace elements necessary to build and sustain health.

Dr. W.A.P. Black, of the British Nutrition Society, says that "Seaweed contains all the elements that have so far been shown to play an important part in the physiological processes of man." The vitamin C content of seaweed is very high — sometimes higher than in oranges. Seaweed has been the only source of vitamin C for many Eskimo tribes and has helped them to survive on an otherwise unhealthful diet. Kelp also contains vitamins B, A, E, K, D and even B_{12}, which is seldom found in foods of vegetable origin. In addition to large amounts of such minerals as calcium, potassium, and chlorine, kelp contains trace minerals such as manganese, copper, silicon, boron, barium, lithium, strontium, zinc, and vanadium. Kelp is extremely rich in all these vital elements because it grows in an ideal environment, with no risk of depletion as it is constantly renewed by nature.

Seaweed is also an excellent source of high quality proteins, which are comparable in biological value to animal proteins.

Seaweed is an essential ingredient in one of the most famous aphrodisiacs — *Bird Nest Soup.* Bird nest soup is prepared from the nest of the sea-swallow. The secret of the aphrodisiac efficacy of bird nest soup is that swallows make their nests from seaweed plants which they glue together with fish spawn. Spawn is rich in phosphorus, and seaweed — with its storehouse of important minerals, particularly iodine — has a rejuvenative and stimulating effect on glandular activity, especially on the thyroid gland, which is responsible for sex drive and libido. Kelp aids in the formation of the thyroid hormone, which regulates the utilization of oxygen by all the cells of the body. Many researchers feel that insufficient oxygenation of cells is at the root of the aging processes. Thus, kelp, or bird nest soup, may be one of the best fountains of youth yet!

Bird nest soup is served in all better Chinese restaurants in the United States, although it is prohibitively expensive. A less expensive, and equally effective way to rejuvenate yourself is to learn from the Japanese and make kelp an essential part of your diet. Kelp is sold in all health food stores in tablet form or granules. It could be added to salads, soups, breads, or vegetable juices. It is an excellent substitute for salt . . . which should be excluded from a health and rejuvenation diet anyway, as you can see from the following.

SALT — A KILLER IN DISGUISE

Perhaps the most important health and rejuvenation secret that comes from Japan concerns salt.

The U.N. sponsored World Health Organization (WHO), reported recently from Japan that it has been statistically demonstrated that the frequency of cancer of the stomach in Japan is definitely related to the quantity of salt consumed by the natives. The more salt in the diet — the more stomach cancers. Thus, salt has been indicted as one of the proven carcinogens.

It is significant, however, that only refined commercial salt has been shown to cause cancer. Where natives use kelp, seawater, or natural unrefined sea salt to season their foods, they enjoy excellent health and avoid stomach cancer.

Cancer is, of course, not the only thing that is caused by excessive consumption of salt. Although beneficial in small amounts, salt is extremely toxic in large doses and is a contributing cause of such disorders as kidney problems, heart and blood vessel conditions, high blood pressure, rheumatic diseases, hair loss, and skin disorders.

Civilized man takes far too much salt with his food. Research has revealed that your daily requirement of salt is between 0.2 and 0.6 grams. This amount of salt can easily be obtained from the foods you eat, provided that you eat predominantly raw, uncooked foods (as you should if you are interested in rejuvenation!). Many people eat as much as 10-15 grams of salt a day. In such amounts, salt becomes a dangerous poison, causing illness and shortening life.

In your rejuvenation diet, keep salt to an absolute minimum. If you use salt, use only natural, unrefined sea salt. Still better, use kelp liberally as a salt substitute. While salt is a life shortener, kelp is one of the best-proved health-building and rejuvenative foods.

As Herbert Spencer said, "the whole secret of prolonging one's life consists in doing nothing to shorten it." And over-indulgence in salt will definitely shorten your life.

8

REJUVENATION SECRETS FROM HUNZA

Hunza, an isolated kingdom in the Himalayas, is known to be a country without disease. Hunza people are also known for their legendary longevity. Many live to be 110 and 125 years of age, and are strong, virile, and active as long as they live, retaining their youthful appearance far into advanced age. Their men have been known to sire children after they reached 100. The *average* life expectancy in Hunza is between 85 and 90 years.

Many investigators have tried to pin down the health and rejuvenation secret of the people of Hunza. The most authoritative and reliable information comes from Dr. Robert McCarrison, who lived among them for seven years. Dr. McCarrison's conclusion was that the traditional diet of the Hunza people was, more than anything else, responsible for their extraordinary health and longevity. Many laymen investigators and authors have visited Hunza since McCarrison, and each one expressed their conclusions as to the Hunzakuts' health and rejuvenation secrets. The last scientific investigator to study the health and longevity records of the Hunza people was my friend, Dr. Karl-Otto Aly, of Sweden. With a large group of Swedish researchers, he stayed in Hunza for several weeks and made a thorough study of their health conditions, their living habits, and their nutritional patterns.

Most investigators point out that in addition to the fact that the Hunza people live a life protected from civilization's hazards — polluted air, water, and soil, and refined, processed foods — the two most important factors in their unusual

health and longevity are:
1. Their high natural carbohydrate-low animal protein diet.
2. The highly mineralized water they drink.

Let's look at these two most important health and rejuvenation secrets from Hunza.

LOW ANIMAL PROTEIN DIET –
HUNZA'S HEALTH AND REJUVENATION
SECRET NUMBER ONE

Dr. Karl-Otto Aly, M.D., is one of the leading biologically and nutritionally oriented doctors in Europe. He is an internationally recognized authority on health and nutrition. In addition to being the director of a large and successful biological clinic in Sweden, he writes and travels extensively, lecturing on health and how it can be built and maintained. A few years ago, he lectured in the United States under the auspices of the National Health Federation.

Dr. Aly made an extensive study of the health conditions and the living habits of the Hunza people during his long stay among them. He examined their birth and death records, spoke to the only physician who lives and practices in the country (who, according to the King of Hunza, "does not have much to do"), examined many natives, and made many tests. Here's what Dr. Aly wrote after his return from Hunza:

"Their daily diet consists even today of natural, poison-free high quality foods, and is mostly vegetarian. The variety of vegetables and fruits guarantees their adequate supply of various minerals, vitamins, and proteins. The fact that Hunzakuts not only survived in their isolated, rugged mountains, but are enjoying such a high level of health and vitality on such a diet, speaks for its inherent superiority."

"According to today's scientific norms and recommendations, the diet of Hunzakuts is utterly protein-deficient, and even deficient in vitamin B_{12}. If we would believe today's orthodox nutritionists, the people of Hunza should have been dead circa 2000 years ago, when they inhabited this isolated river valley and began eating their traditional low animal protein diet. But, apparently not knowing that modern science would not approve of their diet, they fared quite well for over 2000 years. Just like a bumble-bee, which according to all statistical and aerodynamic calculations can't fly, but, being ignorant of the laws of aerodynamics and gravity, flies anyway! Not only did the people of Hunza survive with flying colors, but even today I could not discover a single case of protein deficiency (Kwashiorkor), or anemia and nerve degeneration caused by a B_{12} deficiency."

We are living in an era of the high-protein craze. Some modern nutritionists and doctors, misled by erroneous conclusions of some 19th century scientists and by slanted research paid for by the meat and dairy industries, have been brainwashing us to believe that we must eat "lots of protein" if we wish to be healthy and live long. Disregarding all the empirical evidence to the contrary, they are telling us that not only do we need lots of protein — "the more the better" — but also that we must eat *animal* proteins — meat, fowl, eggs, milk, and fish — if we do not wish to succumb to most horrible diseases. Consequently, we have been filling ourselves up to our ears with proteins. Americans eat more protein than any other people. Also, according to statistics, the United States leads the world in most degenerative diseases, such as cancer, heart disease, arthritis, diabetes, and osteoporosis.

What's wrong? Could it possibly be that modern nutritional scientists have made a mistake — that, perhaps, a high protein diet is not as "good for you" as they believed it would be? Perhaps their tales and scare-stories about kwashiorkor and B_{12} deficiency anemia are not based on scientific facts, but on wishful thinking influenced by their own tastes?

The Hunza example, supported by a growing amount of new nutritional research from around the world, is contradicting and nullifying most of the claims made by the high-animal-protein diet advocates. The latest research shows that the high protein theory was a myth; that most of our present beliefs and conclusions about proteins, our need for them and their function in nutrition *are wrong.* The most recently proven facts about protein, based on the most reliable and authoritative scientific research from independent sources, such as The Max Planck Institute in Germany, The Russian Institute for Nutritional Research, and The International Society for Research on Civilization Diseases and Vital Substances, show:

- That our actual daily requirement of protein is much lower than was believed: not 200, 120, 80, or even 70 grams, as was advocated a decade ago, or 55 grams as recommended in the latest official tables, but only 25 to 30 grams a day!
- That too much protein in the diet is extremely dangerous and can cause many health disturbances and serious diseases.
- That overconsumption of protein can cause a severe deficiency of magnesium and vitamins B_6 and B_3.
- That too much animal protein in the diet contributes to such diseases as arthritis, osteoporosis, heart disease, and cancer. One of the by-products of protein metabolism, ammonia, is considered to be a strong carcinogen.
- That too much protein can cause mental disorders, particularly schizophrenia.
- That too much animal protein in the diet leads to premature aging by causing biochemical imbalance, overacidity in tissues, intestinal putrefaction and constipation, and degeneration of vital organs.

Furthermore, the newest research has established the following extremely important facts, hitherto unknown to science:

1. That the commonly held belief that only animal proteins are complete, and that all vegetable proteins are incomplete, or lacking one or more essential amino acids, is false. Many vegetable sources, such as soybeans, sunflower seeds, almonds, millet, buckwheat, sesame seeds, peanuts, all sprouted seeds and grains, all leafy green vegetables, and potatoes contain complete protein.
2. That vegetable proteins are not only equal to, but they are actually *superior* in biological value to those of animal sources. For example, proteins in potatoes are biologically superior to proteins in meat, eggs, or milk (Max Planck Institute).

3. That raw proteins have higher biological values than cooked proteins. You need only one-half the amount of proteins if you eat raw vegetable proteins instead of animal proteins, which are, as a rule, cooked.

High protein diet — a sure road to premature aging.

High protein propagandists, meat-dairy industries, and protein supplement manufacturers use many tricks to induce you to eat huge amounts of protein: you are made of protein; your hair, your nails, your enzymes, your organs, your hormones — all are made of protein. This is only a half truth. Your hair, nails, and vital organs are not made of protein only, but are made from minerals, trace elements, unsaturated and saturated fatty acids, lecithin . . . *and* proteins!

Another method widely used by high-protein peddlers is preying on the public's gullibility and desire to "look and feel young." They scream, "Stay younger longer with lots of protein, especially meat!" The fact is that heavy meat eating is one of the surest ways to age before your time — physically, sexually, and mentally. The Hunza example illustrates clearly that *it is not a high-protein, but a low-protein diet which has the greatest potential for optimum health and long life.* Their average daily intake of protein is about 30 grams. Many other long-living people in the world, like the Russians, Yukatan Indians, Todas, Abhkazians, Vilcabamba inhabitants, and Bulgarians, are people who eat low-protein diets. Hunzakuts eat meat once a month, at the most. According to a recent study of Dr. S. Magsood Ali, of Pakistan, only 1 percent of the Hunzakuts' protein intake was from animal sources. Bulgarians eat very little meat — perhaps 15 - 20 percent of the average American's consumption. In Russia, only 1½ percent of the total population are vegetarians, while 9 percent of all people who reach 100 years are vegetarians. The healthiest people in Latin America, with the longest life expectancy, are the Yucatan Indians, who never eat meat. Vilcabamba inhabitants in Ecuador show the largest number of centenarians of any place in the world — 1098 for every 100,000 people! According to Dr. Alexander Leaf, M.D., their average protein intake is 35-38 grams a day, and the total caloric intake is only 1200 to 1360 a day. They are almost 100 percent vegetarians. This is something to ponder for those who claim that lots of animal proteins in your diet will keep you younger longer. The opposite is true!

That a high protein diet, particularly a high animal protein diet, is one of the main causes of senility and premature aging has been recently stressed by two leading European biochemists and doctors — Professor Ph. Schwarz, of Frankfurt University, and Dr. Ralph Bircher of Zurich, Switzerland. They reported that the aging processes are triggered by a substance called *amyloid,* a by-product of protein metabolism, which is deposited in connective tissues and causes tissue and organ degeneration. Amyloid, the aging-producing substance, contains a large percentage of the amino acids tryptophan and tyrosine, which are plentiful in animal proteins.

The connection between deposits of amyloid in the tissues and the degenerative diseases and aging processes in man has been known for a long time, but conveniently forgotten in this age of the high protein fad. Famous German pathologist, Dr. Rudolf Virchow, suggested as early as 1854 that amyloid deposits cause degenerative changes and premature aging. Amyloidosis was produced in experimental animals by feeding them high-protein diets.

Now you can see why the Hunza people, in defiance of all the theories of the high-protein cultists, enjoy excellent health and extraordinary longevity on the low-protein diet. Not having read the American health books which expound the virtues of a high-protein diet, they continue to eat their extremely low protein diet (only about 1/3 of the average American's protein intake) and to reap the glorious benefits in the form of total freedom from disease and a long life in youthful vitality.

According to Dr. Alexander Leaf, M.D., who visited Hunza and made an extensive study of their diet as related to their exceptionally long life, the factors mostly responsible for their long life are: 1) their total low-calorie diet (an average of 1900 calories a day) and 2) their predominantly vegetarian diet (only 1 percent of their protein intake comes from animal sources).

What can you learn from the Hunza people regarding proteins? Cut down on all proteins, especially animal proteins. The diet with the greatest potential for optimum health and a long life is a lacto-vegetarian diet with emphasis on vegetables, fruits and seeds, nuts and grains, especially in a sprouted form. Homemade cottage cheese (kvark) and soured milk products can supplement this diet, along with vegetable oils and honey. Meat can be left out completely, or the amount consumed reduced drastically. Overindulgence in protein, especially animal protein, is incompatable with a rejuvenation diet. Remember: People with low-protein diets enjoy the highest life expectancy, while people who eat a high-animal-protein diet enjoy the lowest. The average life expectancy of Eskimos and Lapplanders, who eat very high protein diets, is only 30-35 years.

MINERALIZED WATER –
HUNZA'S HEALTH AND REJUVENATION
SECRET NUMBER TWO

One of America's most popular and knowledgeable nutritionists, Betty Lee Morales, made two visits to Hunza recently, and in the course of a conversation with the Mir (the King of Hunza), had asked him:

"We notice that you serve your Western guests a clear water, while you and your family drink a cloudy looking water. Please tell us the difference."

The Mir's answer reveals one of the most important health and rejuvenation secrets from this land of superior health and perpetual youth:

"Hunza water – the kind that comes down from the glaciers – is the one we here prefer to drink. We *attribute our good health and long life to this water,* which we use both for drinking and for watering our crops. The cloudiness is caused by the minerals and trace minerals picked up as the water flows over many kinds of rocks and stones. The clear water comes from the only well in Karimibad, and, frankly, we keep it active only for our visitors; we never drink that kind ourselves.

"Over at the guest house we set some of this water aside in a glass. After three days, it has not settled at all. Why don't the minerals settle to the bottom?" asked Betty Lee Morales.

"This is the secret, we believe, of the good health our water imparts," answered the Mir. "If the minerals, in microscopic particles, can't settle down in the water, perhaps they are carried into our cells and bone marrow, too. Minerals are a form of metals, I believe, and as metals they may have something to do with transference of energy. In any case, we don't need dentists, and our bones are very strong."*

The erroneous belief that our body can use only organic minerals, and that inorganic minerals (such as those present in so-called hard, mineralized water) are not only useless, but can be harmful, has long ago been disproved. The newest world-wide research clearly shows that inorganic minerals, far from being useless or harmful, are actually essential for man's health. Both organic (as in plants and other foods) and inorganic (as in water and seawater), minerals are needed for the healthy functioning of your body. Extensive research shows that in the areas where people drink hard, mineral-rich water, there is less heart disease, diabetes, tooth decay, and hardening of the arteries. Soft water areas show the greatest incidence of the above conditions (see Chapter 3).

It has been a growing fad in recent years to drink distilled water. While drinking distilled water can be advisable in some rare cases of certain diseases (on a doctor's advice), the regular prolonged use of distilled water is definitely harmful! Man has used natural, mineral-rich water from springs, rivers, and lakes for thousands of years and enjoyed wonderful health. Inorganic minerals in natural waters have always been an integral part of man's environment, and *an essential part of his mineral nutrition is derived from his drinking water.* To deprive yourself of this important mineral nutrition by drinking distilled water can be an extremely dangerous practice.

---

* Betty Lee Morales, "A Visit with the Mir of Hunza", *Let's Live*, April, 1972.

The Hunza example teaches as a good lesson. *Hard, highly-mineralized natural water, far from being harmful, is a very important factor in optimum health and longevity diet.*

In this age of universal water pollution, tap water is seldom fit for drinking, and a growing number of people drink bottled water. Both natural spring water and distilled water are easily obtained. Unless you are fortunate enough to have your own well or spring, make sure you buy the right kind of bottled water — if you wish to avoid the degenerative diseases and premature aging.

9

REJUVENATION SECRETS
from
THE ORIENT

From the East, come two of the most important health and rejuvenation secrets: millet and halvah. Health writers often speak of "miracle foods", "wonder foods", "super foods." Millet and sesame seeds (from which halvah is made) are *true super foods,* which can help you to enjoy better health and stay younger longer.

MILLET

While millet is practically unknown in the United States and is only consumed by a small number of health-minded people (and the birds!) it is the basic grain food in most of the countries in the Near and Far East, China, and Africa. Although it is generally believed that rice is the staple grain of the Chinese people, actually more millet than rice is consumed in China, particularly in the northern parts where it is too cold to grow rice. The Hindu diet is based largely on millet. It is also commonly used in large parts of Africa.

Millet is one of the most nutritious foods known to man. It is the most nutritious of the cereals, possibly sharing this distinction with buckwheat. Many nutritionists believe that the reason why the North Chinese people are generally considered superior in physique to the South Chinese, is because the North Chinese are millet-eating people, while the South Chinese are rice-eating people.

Millet has been used by man for his food longer than any other grain. Pythagoras, over 2500 years ago, praised the nutritional value of millet and advocated its use for his followers as a basis of their diets. As records show, the

Egyptians had consumed millet for thousands of years before Pythagoras. The nutritional value of millet is based on its following virtues:

- Millet is a complete protein food — unique among cereals, which usually are not complete protein foods. Millet contains all the essential amino acids and is comparable in biological protein value to meat or milk. Only one cup of millet meal supplies 34 grams (about a full day's requirement!) of the highest grade proteins.
- Millet is richer in vitamins and minerals than any other grains with the exception of wild rice. According to Professors Osborne and Mendel, millet contains all the essential vitamins and minerals, especially calcium and magnesium, plus all the important trace elements, such as molybdenum.
- Millet is an alkaline food; again, one of the few cereal foods to be in this class. Therefore, even those who suffer from overacidity and related conditions, such as rheumatism, arthritis and diabetes, and consequently cannot use acid-forming grains such as wheat, can eat millet without any discomfort.
- Millet is a complete food in which all nutritional factors — complete proteins, unsaturated fatty acids, lecithin, vitamins, minerals, and carbohydrates — are balanced in ideal proportions. This explains why millet is considered to be one of the very few foods with the capacity to sustain life and good health as an exclusive diet. There are many examples of famines in China, India, and Rumania, during which people lived almost entirely on millet for extended periods of time and remained in good health.

In addition, millet is non-fattening, which cannot be said of most other cereals. This is because millet is an alkali-forming food, and alkalies tend to dissolve and counteract fat building.

If you add to this the fact that millet is also one of the tastiest of all grains, then you can understand why I consider millet to be the king of all cereals, and rejuvenation cereal number one.

How to prepare millet

Buy organically grown millet from your health food store. Most millet grown in the United States comes from North Dakota, where it is normally grown without the aid of sprays and chemical fertilizers (millet grows well even in comparatively poor soils).

Use only hulled millet. Do not be afraid that the hulling of millet removes its nutrients, for it does not. Millet hulls are hard outer cores, and are useless for human consumption. All proteins, vitamins, and minerals are present in hulled millet.

Millet is one of the cereals that is best eaten cooked. Here are two ways to prepare delicious millet cereals.

MILLET CEREAL

1 cup hulled millet
3 - 4 cups water
1/2 tsp. honey
1/2 cup non-instant powdered skim milk (optional)

Rinse millet in warm water and drain. Place in a pan of water, mixed with powdered skim milk and heat the mixture to the boiling point. Then simmer for ten minutes, stirring occasionally to prevent sticking and burning. Remove from heat and let stand for a half hour or more. Serve with milk, honey, cold-pressed vegetable oil, or butter.

MILLET CEREAL (Low-heat oven method)

Place all the ingredients, as above, in a pan with a tight cover. Use heat-proof utensil, such as pyrex, earthenware, or stainless steel. Place in an electric oven turned on low: 200 degrees F, or less if possible. Leave for 3 to 4 hours, even more if desired, but the cereal will be ready to eat in about 3 hours.

This is a superior method of preparing millet cereal because of the low temperature, which makes the nutrients of millet, particularly the proteins, more assimilable. Serve in the same manner as described in the first recipe.

HALVAH

While millet has been used by man longer than any other grain, sesame seeds have been used longer than any other seed, going back to the earliest stages of civilization. Cultivated by man for thousands of years, sesame is named in many ancient writings as a special rejuvenation food. It is used widely in Africa and in the Middle and Far East. In India and China, sesame is a staple food. Armenian Turks use it in a liquid form called *Matahini,* which is considered to be a respected rejuvenator of mental and physical capacities and endurance. In Israel, Turkey, and Arabian countries, a candy made from sesame seeds and honey — Halvah — is very popular. The women of ancient Babylonia used halvah to enhance their sex appeal and to restore the virility of their men.

Halvah is available even in the United States, mostly from old-country type markets and delicatessens, and also from health food stores. Health food stores also sell a butter-like spread made from sesame seeds, called *Tahini.*

While millet is the King of Cereals, sesame in the King of Seeds. Sesame seeds are extremely nutritious. They are richer in calcium than milk, cheese, or nuts. Their protein content is 19 percent to 28 percent higher than that of meat, and sesame protein is of very high value, comparable in quality to the protein in meat. Sesame seeds are especially good sources of the important amino acid methionine, which is otherwise scarce in proteins of vegetable source.

Sesame seeds are also very rich in unsaturated fatty acids — up to 55 percent of the seed is oil. They are also rich in B-vitamins: niacin, inositol and choline, and vitamin E.

Both millet and sesame, by the way, are excellent sources of lecithin, an organic phosphorized fat which is a chief constituent of brain and nerve tissues, and an essential component of semen. Lecithin is an effective aid in keeping your blood vessels free from cholesterol deposits. It is also vitally important for the proper function of important glands that are to a great extent responsible for your looking and feeling young: pituitary, pineal and sex glands.

Sesame seeds, in combination with honey (halvah), become

a very important rejuvenation food. French doctors who investigated the popular belief that halvah is a powerful aphrodisiac, found that the rejuvenative property of halvah can be scientifically explained. Sesame seeds have abundant magnesium and potassium, and honey is rich in aspartic acid, one of the amino acids. Some doctors have used a very similar prescription formula — the potassium and magnesium salts of aspartic acid — to treat women with "the housewife syndrome", or chronic fatigue, insomnia, and lethargy in lovemaking — 87 percent responded with a startling improvement in condition. Aspartic acid is an important rejuvenative factor, particularly for sexual rejuvenation.

Sesame seeds are sold in most health food stores. They can be used in many ways to enhance your diet. Sprinkle them on cereals, salads, mix or blend them in drinks, or make your own homemade halvah.

Here is the recipe for it:

HALVAH*

1 cup sesame seeds

2 tsp. coagulated, natural honey

Grind sesame seeds in an electric seed grinder. Pour sesame meal into a large cup and knead honey into it with a large spoon until honey is well mixed in and halvah acquires the consistency of hard dough. Serve it as it is, or make small balls and roll in whole sesame seeds, shredded coconut, sunflower seeds, or wheat germ — and enjoy one of the finest and best tasting health and rejuvenation foods in the world!

The Romans had an old custom of giving soldiers an emergency ration — cakes made of sesame seeds and honey. Experience had convinced them that man could walk farther and survive longer on this ration than on any other food of equal weight.

---

* Note: Commercial halvah is made with sugar and eggwhite, which is used as binding agent. I have formulated this simple recipe, using only sesame seeds and honey. It holds together well, especially if sesame seeds are ground very fine and hard, coagulated honey is used. And it's simply super-delicious! Make sure, however, that the sesame seeds are 100 percent fresh, not rancid. They turn stale and rancid in about 6 months after they are harvested.

10

Rejuvenation Secrets
from
MEXICO

Mexico is one of the countries in which I have had the opportunity to travel and study the most. My clinical work was done largely in our Mexican Spa, where I had an opportunity to observe the results of many rejuvenative therapies employed at the clinic.

Herbal medical science is highly advanced in Mexico. It has ancient traditions, stemming from the extensive use of herbs for healing and rejuvenation by Mayan, Aztec, and other native Indians. While the popularity of herbal medicines has declined during this century in the rest of the world, in Mexico herbs are used by everyone just as much now as they ever were. Every market place features many *yerbalistas,* who are well educated in the medicinal properties of Mexican herbs. I dare say that even today more people in Mexico use medicinal herbs for healing than chemical drugs from *farmacias.*

By living in Mexico for many years, I also discovered that the traditional Mexican diet features several powerful health and longevity factors. Let's look at these first.

PAPAYA, LIME, AND CHILI

The Mexican contribution to my international list of health-building and rejuvenating foods are three foods which are used by the Mexicans as staples in their traditional diet: papaya, lime, and chili.

Papaya is a tropical fruit, which grows abundantly in Mexico, in the south and as far north as Mazatlan. It is rich in the enzyme *papain,* which is an effective digestive aid. Papain helps break down protein into amino acids and makes them easily assimilable. Papaya is also extremely rich in vitamins — particularly vitamin C — and minerals.

Mexicans eat papaya as a dessert, especially after a protein-rich meal. This is an excellent habit, since it can be truthfully said that *we are not what we eat,* but *what we assimilate.* Papaya helps the digestive tract to digest and assimilate protein-rich foods more effectively.

Papaya is also an excellent cleansing food, with many remarkable therapeutic properties. My good friend, Dr. B. Lytton-Bernard, has used papaya and papaya juice to treat many conditions — including digestive disorders, arthritis, obesity, and kidney diseases — with remarkable results.

Papayas are sold in most supermarkets in the United States. They are usually imported from Mexico or Hawaii. Health food stores also sell papaya juice, canned papaya, papaya pulp, and digestive tablets containing papain.

Lime is another digestion-promoting food that Mexicans use liberally. In fact, in the traditional Mexican diet, limes are used with every conceivable food or drink: Mexicans serve cut limes with any kind of order in restaurants; they squeeze lime on all fruits and vegetables, including papaya; they squeeze it into juices and drinks, including beer and tequila; and they squeeze lime juice on meat, fish, and any other kind of prepared dish. Lime is also considered to be one of the best medicines, especially for colds, skin diseases, stomach disorders, dysentery ("turista") or for disinfection and healing of fresh wounds and scratches.

The medicinal value of lime is well documented by extensive research. It is a powerful antiseptic. It is also anti-scorbutic: that is, it will help to prevent disease and will assist in cleansing the system of impurities. Lime or lemon is also a wonderful stimulant to the liver; it dissolves uric acid crystals in the tissues; and it is an excellent help in the digestion of food. It is rich in digestive enzymes and its acid property helps to create an acid condition in the stomach, which is necessary for protein and mineral digestion. Lemon and lime juice are specific in the treatment of such conditions as asthma, colds, liver complaints, scurvy, dysentery, fevers, and digestive problems.

In recent years, the addition of apple cider vinegar to the diet has become very popular in the United States. As people grow older, their digestion tends to become sluggish, mostly because of the diminished secretion of hydrochloric acid in the stomach. Apple cider vinegar, although it does not substitute for the hydrochloric acid entirely, creates an acid condition in the stomach and helps to improve digestion, especially of proteins and minerals. In Mexico, lime juice is used for the same purpose. In my experience, lime or lemon juice in small amounts is preferable to apple cider vinegar, as it has, in addition to its beneficial acids, many important vitamins, minerals, and enzymes.

Finally, *chili* is another Mexican contribution to better health and longer life. Nowhere in the world is chili consumed to the extent that it is in Mexico. As with lime juice, chili powder is sprinkled on virtually everything, including oranges, apples, mangoes, and watermelon. It is also added to practically every cooked food, and not in just microscopic amounts to spike or enhance the natural flavors in food, but in such huge amounts that most non-Mexicans have to gasp for air and water after a single bite of any traditional Mexican food.

Mexicans use many kinds of chilies, some mild, like our regular green or red peppers, some so strong that a mere rub on the skin will produce a blister. The strong, tiny chili-peppers are used mostly for cooking and making salza, a Mexican dressing prepared with chili, tomatoes, garlic, and onions. Milder chilies are often eaten raw in salads. Cayenne, or red pepper, is the most commonly used chili throughout Mexico.

Can these strong peppers be healthful? While mustard and white and black pepper, which are commonly used in the United States, are definitely harmful, toxic, and irritating to the delicate linings of the stomach and bowels, cayenne pepper or chili is extremely beneficial and soothing. It has many wonderful medicinal properties. It stimulates circulation, it helps digestion by stimulating the production of enzymes and hydrochloric acid in the stomach, it exerts a beneficial, stimulating action on kidneys, spleen, and pancreas, and it is considered to be a powerful general tonic and stimulant. If you ask an average Mexican why he is so healthy, he will inevitably answer: chili.

By the way, chilies are extremely rich in vitamins, minerals, and enzymes, especially in vitamin C.

My conclusion is that chili has definite health-promoting and age-retarding properties if used in moderate amounts.

MEXICAN REJUVENATING HERBS

Herbs are used in every country and by every race for healing and rejuvenating purposes, and have been so used throughout the ages. Mexico has many potent herbs that are used for healing disease. Since this book deals primarily with rejuvenation, two special rejuvenating herbs come to my mind: damiana and sarsaparilla.

Damiana is mostly known and highly regarded as an aphrodisiac. It is used widely, not only in Mexico, but in most Central and South American countries. It is sold by every Mexican village or town herbalist.

There are many kinds of damiana. The kind mostly used in Mexico is known botanically as *Turnera Aphrodisiaca.* It grows in California, all over Mexico, and in Central and South America. Damiana grown in Baja California is considered to be the most potent. Damiana grows as a shrub or small tree, with small narrow leaves. The leaves are dried and used mostly as tea, which has a slightly bitter taste.

Damiana is used mostly as an aphrodisiac. It is an old remedy for sexual impotence. It is reported to strengthen and enhance the function of reproductive organs. Damiana is known to be a tonic for the nerves and is used in cases of mental and physical exhaustion. It is also a stimulant to the kidneys and increases the flow of urine.

Damiana is prepared as most herb teas: 1 tsp. of dried leaves to 1 cup of water. Pour boiling water over the leaves and let stand and steep for 15 minutes. Take one cup twice a day. Most health food stores and herb stores in the United States sell damiana.

Sarsaparilla is another Mexican rejuvenative herb. Sarsaparilla is a tropical plant which grows mostly in Honduras, Mexico, Jamaica, and Equador, but also in China and Japan. The botanical name is *Smilax Medica* or *Smilax Regalii.* It is an evergreen herb, and the root is the only part used for medicinal purposes.

Sarsaparilla is considered to be a powerful blood purifier and also is used for such conditions as chronic rheumatism, skin disorders, psoriasis, general weakness, and sexual impotence. It is considered to be a potent antidote for the toxic effects of any strong poison.

But, for the purpose of this presentation, the most important fact about sarsaparilla is that it is a potent natural source of male and female sex hormones, which are involved in keeping the body and mind young. American and Mexican scientists discovered — independently of each other — that sarsaparilla roots contain *testosterone,* a male sex hormone. And recently it was discovered that sarsaparilla also contains *progesterone,* the female sex hormone. Even *cortin* — one of the adrenal hormones — was found in sarsaparilla.

In recent times, therefore, Mexican and South American pharmaceutical companies have been manufacturing male and female sex hormone tablets from natural hormones isolated from sarsaparilla.

It is generally considered that the strength of the endocrine glands, and particularly the sex glands, and their ability to produce sufficient hormones, is directly related to the general vitality and healthy functioning of the body. Sexual virility largely determines man's youthfulness, health, vitality, and longevity. Likewise, plentiful sex hormone production in the female makes her look, feel, and act young. The decline in sex hormone production results in gradual aging and decreased life span. Therefore, sarsaparilla can be listed as one of the most important of natural rejuvenators. It can help to supply the missing hormones and bring the spark of youth back into your life.

Sarsaparilla roots (the red Honduras sarsaparilla is considered the most potent) are boiled in water for 15 to 30 minutes, and the decoction is drunk as a tea twice a day. Use one ounce of the root to one pint of water.

Perhaps this will be the proper place to give a few other herbal secrets, especially for female rejuvenation. The aging processes in the female are accelerated after menopause, when the glandular activity slows down and sex hormone deficiencies, especially the deficiency of estrogen, will manifest itself. Many women drug themselves with the synthetic hormone, estrogen, to slow down the aging processes. This can be very dangerous, as it is well known that taking synthetic estrogen can lead to the development of cancer. There are several good sources of natural estrogen, which is totally harmless: licorice, unicorn roots, falce unicorn, and elder flowers. Use them like any other herbs — as teas.

11

Rejuvenation Secrets
from
CHINA

Since the communist take-over several decades ago, China has been out of contact with the rest of the world. The bamboo curtain is now open, and many Western travelers are anxiously looking East in hopes of learning something from this, perhaps, the oldest civilization in the world.

Already we are astounded at some of the medical secrets that are coming out of China. Acupuncture is one of them. This 5,000-year-old Chinese art of healing has amazed the entire Western medical world. "It may well be . . .that the latter half of the 20th Century will one day be called the Golden Age of Acupuncture", wrote the *New York Times.* Western doctors have learned that the Chinese technique of inserting needles at various points in the body can have dramatic curative effects on a wide range of ailments extending from headaches and muscular pains to serious heart disease, arthritis, diabetes, and other disorders.

But even while China was securely behind the bamboo curtain, rejuvenation-conscious Westerners had continuous contact with the Eastern art of rejuvenation through the use of famous oriental herbs — notably ginseng, and gotu-kola. These two herbs, used in China and its close neighbors Manchuria and Korea for thousands of years, are credited with remarkable rejuvenative properties.

GINSENG

Ginseng is the most famous and the most potent rejuvenating plant. The roots of the ginseng bear a remarkable resemblance to the shape and form of man: this is why the Chinese called the plant, *ginseng*, or "man-plant".

Ginseng has been used by 500 million Chinese and many more millions of other Orientals for over 5,000 years as an effective aphrodisiac, rejuvenator, revitalizer, and cure-all for a variety of ills. Ginseng has been used widely even in the United States in recent years, but it was almost banned recently by FDA action. The FDA took this drastic action on the grounds that ginseng is totally useless and worthless for the purposes claimed. Such criticism of ginseng was expressed by many even before the FDA action, claiming that ginseng does not produce the anticipated results. If ginseng did not produce genuine results, if its power was based on nothing more than sheer superstition, don't you think man would have discarded it long before now? You may be able to fool 50 million Frenchmen, but you can hardly fool 500 million Chinese! In spite of the fact that ginseng is very expensive in China — valued almost at the price of gold — it is bought and used by millions of people. In some cases, the very poor people sell their last possessions to buy this rejuvenative herb.

Is the reputation of ginseng based on ignorance and superstition, or can it be substantiated by scientific research?

The Russian Institute of Experimental Medicine made an extensive study of ginseng and its claimed medicinal and rejuvenating properties. They discovered that ginseng grows only in radioactive soil, and that the roots of the plant itself contain many radioactive properties. In fact, this radioactive property of ginseng helps the collectors of the wild ginseng to locate the plant. The ginseng plant emits its radioactive rays, which are evidenced by a distinct glow at night. Ginseng hunters go out during the night and shoot colored arrows at the glowing plants. The next day, they locate the plants marked by the arrows and dig the roots.

Russian researchers also have found that the claims the Orientals were making about ginseng were true: it strengthens the heart, revitalizes the nervous system, increases hormone production, and stimulates cell growth and activity. After the results of this research were reported to the Russian

Government, it immediately ordered the establishment of huge plantations of ginseng in Southern Siberia. Russians also buy most of the ginseng produced in North Korea, while most of the ginseng produced in South Korea is sold to the United States.

Ginseng grows wild in some parts of central United States. There are also many plantations, both here and in other parts of the world, where ginseng is grown commercially. The plant must be at least 6 years old before the roots can be collected.

The bulk of all ginseng sold in the United States comes from Korea and China. Ginseng is sold in all health food stores in powder, tablet, or capsule form. It is also available as a whole root or packaged in tea bags.

HYDROCOTYLE ASIATICA MINOR (GOTU-KOLA)

Hydrocotyle Asiatica Minor is another well-known rejuvenator. It is a small plant that grows only in certain jungle districts of the Oriental tropics.

It was popularized by the renowned Chinese scholar and herbalist, Professor Li Chung Yun, who lived to be 265 years of age. Don't laugh! Professor Li Chung Yun's age is well documented. Being a world-famous scholar, he was in the public eye for over 200 years. At the age of 100, he was awarded by the Chinese government a special Honor Citation for extraordinary services to his country. This document is available in existing archives. For over 150 years after the award, the Professor was visited by countless Western scholars and students. It is reported that he gave a series of 28 lectures at the University of Sinkiang when he was over 200 years old.

His life spanned four centuries – 16th, 17th, 18th, and 19th. He enjoyed excellent health, outlived 23 wives, and kept his own natural teeth and hair. Those who saw him at the age of 200 testified that he did not appear much older than a man in his fifties. Professor Li Chung Yun attributed his longevity to his life-long vegetarian diet and the regular use of rejuvenating herbs; plus – may I add, an important plus — to his "inward calm". He used gotu-kola and ginseng daily in the form of tea.

British, French, and Ceylonese researchers, who made studies and clinical tests on Hydrocotyle Asiatica Minor, agree that the plant contains an unknown vitamin, which they termed "vitamin X", or the "youth vitamin". This new vitamin, they say, has a rejuvenating effect on the brain cells and on the endocrine glands. The French government was so impressed by the research on the rejuvenative properties of this plant, that it established several large plantations and experimental research stations in Algeria.

Hydrocotyle Asiatica Minor is available in health food stores, both in pure form, or as an ingredient in an herbal blend called Fo-Ti-Tieng.

The effectiveness of these Oriental rejuvenation herbs is attributed to the fact that they have a stimulating effect on all vital body functions by keeping endocrine and sex glands in peak working condition far into advanced age, and by increasing the production of life-giving hormones, which are the actual "fountains of youth". They also exert an energizing effect on nerve and brain functions and keep blood free from age-causing toxins. Well, if they can do only a fraction of all this they can rightfully be called the "Herbal Fountains of Youth".

Note: There has been much confusion regarding *Fo-ti-tieng.* Some writers claim that Fo-ti-tieng is an herb (as did even this writer earlier, misled by unreliable sources of information). Actually, Fo-ti-tieng is a trade name for an herbal formula made from three different herbs, one of which is *Hydrocotyle Asiatica Minor.*

12

Rejuvenation secrets
from
PITCAIN ISLAND

"From where?" I hear your perplexed question. Even the real veteran health book readers, for whom Hunza is a household word, have, in all probability, never heard of Pitcairn Island.

Pitcairn Island is located in the South Pacific, just below the Tropic of Capricorn, south-east of Tahiti. In 1789, the mutineers of the legendary pirated British armed transport, *Bounty,* led by Fletcher Christian, established an utopian commune on this remote Pacific island, which has been recently stirring much interest among the modern longevity and health researchers. Although the total population of Pitcairn Island has never reached over 233 (and now, mostly due to emigration, has dwindled to 73), the island has lured several investigators and scientists who were impressed by the exceptional health and longevity of these seventh-generation descendants of nine British navymen and their brown Tahitian concubines.

American physician, Dr. David Gibson, of Grand Prairie, who visited Pitcairn Island recently and made a thorough examination and study of their health condition, says, "It would be difficult to find a comparable population anywhere in the world as healthy, robust, and physically fit as these people." He has found that "apart from some minor surgical procedures, there really isn't much to do" there. Although life expectancy studies have never been made on the Pitcairners, most observers have found that the average age of death is in the mid or late seventies — this in spite of the unusual hazards posed in daily life on the island, and that one in every five Pitcairners die by accident at sea, in falls from cliffs, or in hunting mishaps.

Ian Ball, U.S. correspondent for the *Daily Telegraph* of London and the author of the immensely popular book, *Pitcairn: Children of Mutiny* (Little, Brown and Company, 380 pp., $8.95), has spent much time on Pitcairn Island and has made a thorough study of the history, the living and eating habits, and the health condition of the people there. He writes,". . . without question, (they) are the most physically robust society I have ever encountered."

Dr. Gibson was amazed at the youthful vigor and stamina demonstrated by the "old" Pitcairners. Men well over seventy scramble up rope ladders to the decks of ships like only twenty-year-olds elsewhere might do.

When these and other researchers try to pinpoint the actual causes of the exceptional health and longevity of the Pitcairners, they invariably list their diet as the most important cause. Partly as a result of the tight isolation from the "civilized" world, partly because of the sheer availability of the foods, but mainly as a result of the dietary laws of their religion, these human relics of the *Bounty* saga live on a diet which most modern nutritionists have found to be the ideal program for optimum health and long life. At the end of the last century, *all* Pitcairners were converted to the Seventh-Day Adventist faith. Consequently, they are basically vegetarians, the staples of their diet being the abundance of delicious fruits, berries, and vegetables that grow on their island. They do eat some fish, following the injunction in Leviticus to eat only "whatsoever hath fins and scales in the waters", avoiding completely cray fish and shell fish, which abound in Pitcairn waters.

Needless to say, they do not drink or smoke, and most do not use tea or coffee. Homemade fruit drinks and juices are their staple drinks — pineapple juice, wild strawberry juice, orange juice, etc. Dairy products and milk are almost non-existent. All attempts to introduce dairy farming to the island have failed — the cows kept falling off the cliffs. With the exception of imported canned butter, the islanders use hardly any dairy products.

PITCAIRNERS' HEALTH AND LONGEVITY
SECRET NUMBER ONE

As I studied the various living and eating habits of the Pitcairners, trying to pinpoint the prime cause of their superior health and vitality and exceptional longevity, I have uncovered one factor, which I learned from my teacher, Are Waerland, 30 years ago, but which has been somewhat forgotten in this the start-the-day-with-a-hearty-protein-breakfast era. Pitcairners eat their breakfast at noon. Although they start their day at sunrise, or about 5 A.M. and do all kinds of heavy physical labor and activity all morning, they do not eat any solid protein foods until the late breakfast at midday. They start their day with a large mug of pure well water, and then snack on fresh fruits now and then as the morning passes. This practice is of tremendous importance for their health and vitality, as you will soon see.

It is appalling how many of our nutrition advisors recommend eating a large, protein-rich breakfast, as soon as you get out of bed in the morning. This is contrary to all the scientific and empirical evidence that I could uncover during more than a quarter of a century of nutrition research.

During the night, from about 11 P.M. to 5 A.M., your digestive, assimilative, and restorative systems are busy at work, while your eliminative system is at rest. The morning hours from about 5 A.M. to 11 A.M., constitute a period of elimination, when the bloodstream is heavily charged with the waste products of metabolism carried out during the night, and the eliminative organs are doing their job of cleansing the system of impurities and toxins — through the skin, through the lungs, and through the kidneys and alimentary canal. "Morning breath" is just one indication of such elimination. Lack of appetite in the early morning is another. Eating a large breakfast as soon as you get up will disrupt this cleansing process and interrupt the elimination. What your body needs in the early morning is plenty of fresh air, lots of liquids, fresh juicy fruits, and vigorous physical work or exercise to help your body complete its cleansing and eliminating process. Then, but not before, you are ready for breakfast.

Paul Bragg, a veteran health builder, has a good way of putting it. He says, "you must earn your breakfast." So, he goes for a long walk, swims, or does heavy exercise in the morning before he is ready for food. This is how it should be. This is how *all* "natural" people — the natives known for their excellent health — always do. They get up early in the morning, normally "with the sun", and immediately go to their heavy chores: feeding the animals or taking them to the pasture, milking the cows, working the garden or fields, fishing or hunting — or whatever their particular work or life style is. For women it is usually work around the house, preparing the breakfast, baking bread, cleaning the house, etc., etc. Then — *several hours later* — after hard work and plenty of perspiration, they are ready for breakfast. This routine is followed by all healthy natives everywhere: In Hunza, in Bulgaria, in Russia, in Scandinavia, by North, Central, and South American Indians *as well as by Pitcairners.*

To eat a large, protein-rich breakfast right after you've gotten out of bed and when you really are not hungry, is to do yourself a great disservice. This routine is a sure road to premature aging, impaired health, and disease.

Yet, this is exactly what most of our misinformed "authorities" advise us to do. You may not believe me, but I have heard it with my own ears. After a lecture, given by one of those hearty-protein-breakfast advocates, a rather obese lady said to the lecturer, "But, I don't feel hungry in the morning!" To which the lecturer replied: "Don't wait until you get hungry. Eat a large breakfast of liver, steak, eggs, and milk, and you won't get hungry during your working hours."

"Breakfast as a king, lunch as a prince, and dine as a pauper" is a false slogan, contrived by our misled and confused scientists. There are all kinds of *theories* regarding eating and drinking — when you should or shouldn't eat or drink — *theories invented by scientists.* To answer the question for yourself *when* should *you* eat or drink, you don't need scientists or their theories. *Nature* has provided a built-in mechanism within your brain which will tell you unmistakably when you should eat or drink. *You should eat when you are hungry, and drink when you are thirsty.* Contrariwise, you should *never drink when you are not thirsty nor eat when you are not hungry.* Most people are just not hungry at five or six in the morning when they just get out of bed, and before they leave for work. To eat a huge protein-rich breakfast at such a time is to work against your body's own timetable and its requirements. This can seriously endanger your health.

Follow the example of the Pitcairners — drink water or herb tea the first thing in the morning, then an hour or two later snack on fresh, juicy fruit, and eat a hearty breakfast at 11:00 or noon — and see what a difference it will make in the way you feel! To achieve optimum health and long life, you have to work with nature — and its own timetable — not against it.

13

REJUVENATION SECRETS
FROM
AMERICA

As could be expected, the American contribution to the rejuvenation secrets comes in pill form — vitamins, minerals, and food supplements. Since we are more youth-oriented than any other people, a great deal of our attention has been directed not so much towards finding the ways of improving health and preventing the aging processes, as to preserving the appearance of youth. Since Americans are also extremely drug- or pill-oriented, our "youth researchers" and "youth doctors" are trying to find the secret of youth in a single vitamin tablet or other food substance; a fountain of youth in a glass of miracle juice, or a little gelatin capsule that will perform the wonder of rejuvenation.

I am happy to report that there are many vitamins, enzymes, minerals, trace elements, and other food substances that do indeed possess rejuvenative properties and can help prevent the aging processes or even reverse them. One of the researchers who was interested in the prospect of prolongation of life, Dr. Paul de Kruif, says that vitamins are "potent chemicals that will help stretch out your span of productive vitality. We now know that the time to try to push back senility is before we're old in years." Stressing that nutritional deficiencies may be the main cause of premature aging, he continues, "What we eat — while seemingly adequate — may mean the premature aging of many of us. But by using chemical knowledge now available, this premature aging can be reversed." Many other researchers feel that in the "chemical knowledge", or in the nutritive chemicals — vitamins, minerals, etc. – may be hidden the true secret of extended youth. Let's look at some of these.

VITAMIN E

Of all the vitamins, vitamin E is the rejuvenation vitamin number one. This vitamin has been credited with being a miracle youth, virility, and vitality vitamin – a vitamin which can reverse the aging processes and keep you younger longer.

One of the leading American experts on aging – its causes, prevention, and cure – is Dr. Aloys L. Tappel, a biochemist at the University of California, and professor of Food Science and Technology at Davis College. Dr. Tappel says that "Aging is due to the process of oxidation." He writes:

"Aging of our bodies appears to be influenced by an intracellular tug of war going on between two factors acting upon a third: intensity and duration of radiation-like effects: polyunsaturated lipids upon which they act, and the vitamin E available to protect them from excessive destruction."

Dr. Tappel says that as we become older, the oxygenation of our cells is diminished, and because of increased oxidation, certain substances, called *free radicals,* are formed within our cells. These free radicals have a destructive effect on normal cell metabolism, causing damage and contributing to the aging processes. "Perhaps the reason some people look older than their years is that they have been more vulnerable to this damage than those who don't show their age," says Dr. Tappel.

Dr. Tappel's prescription for preventing premature aging is vitamin E. Vitamin E is the most powerful natural anti-oxidant. Dr. Tappel says: "in normal humans, vitamin E, contained in unsaturated vegetable fat, acts to prevent the formation of free radicals and serves as a built-in protection against accelerated aging."

By the way, vitamin E deficiency also causes the formation of a pigment, ceroid, which is thought to be part of aging.

Since our typical American diet is grossly deficient in vitamin E, supplementing it with extra vitamin E in capsule form would be one of the best things you could do for yourself to prevent premature aging, extend life, and stay younger longer. The best natural sources of vitamin E are whole grains, seeds, and nuts, and cold-pressed vegetable oils. Refined foods, such as white flour or bread or processed oils, do not contain enough vitamin E to keep you young, because most of the vitamin E in them has been removed or destroyed in processing.

Vitamin E in capsule form is sold in all health food stores and drug stores. Most doctors recommend doses up to 600 IU as perfectly safe. Older people can take twice as much. Those who suffer from serious diseases should consult their doctors regarding the proper dosage.

Another noted scientist who believes that vitamin E can help to control or even reverse the aging processes, is Dr. Hans Selye, of the University of Montreal. Dr. Selye is the author of the famous stress theory: that all diseases, including premature aging, are caused by stresses which the weakened body is unable to counteract. Vitamin E is one of our basic anti-stress vitamins. It increases the body's resistance to stresses by improving circulation, strengthening the heart, preventing oxidation, and increasing the oxygenation of all tissues and cells. Dr. Selye tells how in animal studies he was able to cause all signs and symptoms of "old age" by deliberately witholding vitamin E from the test animals. Conversely, in the other group of test animals, life and youth was prolonged through the use of vitamin E.

Since vitamin E is also one of the truly miraculous, health-building, and health-restoring substances and helps to save lives by favorably influencing such conditions as heart disease, diabetes, arthritis, arteriosclerosis, varicose veins, ulcers, etc., it must be considered to be one of the most important life-prolongators and rejuvenators. Vitamin E is also a potent rejuvenator of male and female fertility and virility. It has a strong regenerative and stimulating effect on all sexual and reproductive functions. It can prevent miscarriages and spontaneous abortions; it increases fertility of both the male and female; it can restore virility in impotent men and banish frigidity in women. Although you may have heard repeatedly the official medical line that "there is absolutely no evidence" that vitamin E is a sex rejuvenator, there are dozens of reliable clinical studies from around the world which show that vitamin E indeed can do all of the things mentioned above. By improving and regenerating the functions of your sex glands, vitamin E can definitely help you to stay younger longer.

VITAMIN C

As I stressed in Chapter One, many scientists believe that one of the basic causes of premature aging is the degenerative processes in collagen, the intercellular cement which holds the cells together. This deterioration in collagen is largely caused by a vitamin C deficiency. Physiological changes in collagen, caused by a deficiency of vitamin C, lead to such symptoms as wrinkles, flabbiness, and skin discolorations, in addition to adversely affecting all the metabolic processes and speeding up the aging process.

This has been clearly shown by Dr. W.J. McCormick's work. Also, Dr. Tappel stresses, in addition to vitamin E, vitamin C can help to retard the aging processes by improving and strengthening the cellular and collagen integrity. Dr. Tapple recommends supplementing the diet with large doses of vitamin C.

A Japanese researcher, Dr. M. Higuchi, recently reported that his studies show a definite relationship between vitamin C levels in the diet and hormone production of the sex glands. He says that older people, particularly, need larger amounts of vitamin C to assure adequate sex hormone production.

Vitamin C is vitally involved in all the functions of your body. It is our most potent anti-toxin. It helps your body to protect itself against every stress and every condition threatening your health. Since aging processes are often associated with various conditions of diminished health, vitamin C becomes an important life prolongator. By improving cell breathing, vitamin C prevents the premature aging of cells. It also has a beneficial stimulating effect on adrenal glands, helping them in hormone production, particularly in production of cortisone. "You are as young as your glands", believe many scientists. Vitamin C helps your glands to work at the peak of their capacity and keep you younger longer.

A rejuvenation program should include large doses of vitamin C — up to 5000 mg. a day.

VITAMIN A

It has been established by research that the oxygenation of the tissues is enhanced by a combination of vitamins E and A. Vitamin A increases the permeability of blood capillaries. The capillaries carry oxygen and other nutritive substances to every cell of your body. The more permeable these capillary walls, the more oxygen can be delivered to the cells. Thus, vitamin A is a third vitamin (in addition to E and C) that can improve cell oxygenation; and efficient cell oxygenation is the ultimate secret of perpetual youth.

Vitamin A also helps keep your skin youthful at any age, by preventing drying of the skin and keeping it free from blemishes.

Jheri Redding, noted cosmetologist, says that by taking 100,000 units of vitamin A each day you can extend your life span by 10 years.

Two scientists from Columbia University, Drs. H.C. Sherman and Oswald A. Roels, demonstrated that vitamin A helps to prevent premature aging and increases life expectancy. It regulates the stability of tissue in cell wells — cell membranes break down when there is a lack of vitamin A. Vitamin A is also essential for the health of all mucous linings and membranes in the body.

The best natural sources of vitamin A are carrots, tomatoes, and green leafy vegetables. Fish liver oils are the richest natural source. Vitamin A capsules are sold in all health food stores. Rejuvenative doses are 50,000 to 100,000 U.S.P. units a day. There are those who say that large doses of vitamin A can be toxic when taken for prolonged periods of time. It would be wise, therefore, to make 2-3 week intervals every few months if you take doses larger than 50,000. Dr. Kurt Donsbach, noted nutritionist, says that he has been taking 150,000 units daily for years without any adverse effects. As for myself, I have been taking 100,000 units daily for at least four years without interruption, without noticing any side effects. Of course, I also take large doses of practically every other vitamin known. All vitamins are synergistic in their action: that is, they are more effective when taken simultaneously.

Note: If you suffer from any serious illness, or are doubtful about the proper dosage of vitamins and supplements, have a nutritionally oriented doctor prescribe the most suitable dosage *for you.*

B-COMPLEX VITAMINS

As I said, *all* vitamins are important in the overall program of keeping healthy and staying young. In this chapter, I mention only a few which have been proven to be scientific rejuvenators or life prolongators.

From the B-vitamin complex, which includes over twenty different vitamins, specific vitamins that are involved in keeping you young are:

- *Thiamine (B$_1$)* is called the age-fighting vitamin. It protects the heart, it stimulates brain action, and is indispensible for the health of the entire nervous system. B$_1$ helps the pituitary gland to keep sexual desires normal.

- *Niacin.* According to Dr. Abram Hoffer, world's foremost authority on the therapeutic uses of niacin, heart attacks (our greatest killer), strokes, and physical and mental senility can be prevented by large doses of niacin. He recommends 3000 mg. a day as a regular dose for old, senile people. He claims that a good diet, plenty of vitamins and supplements, and large doses of niacin will extend life by 10 to 20 years.

- *Pantothenic acid* is of specific importance to women who wish to delay the onset of menopause. It also protects against every form of stress, increases cortisone production, helps to fight infection, and speeds recovery from ill health. It is also known to help restore color to gray hair.

- *Pangamic acid (B$_{15}$).* Vitamin B$_{15}$ increases the body's tolerance to lowered oxygen supply; thus, it is complementary to the action of the rejuvenative vitamins

E, C, and A, which increase the oxygen supply to the tissues. B_{15} is of particular importance now, in the time of universal air pollution. The most age-producing substance in the polluted air is carbon monoxide, which prevents oxygen from being absorbed by the lungs. Vitamin B_{15} counteracts the effects of carbon monoxide.

- *PABA and Folic Acid.* These two B-vitamins are reported to be specifically involved in keeping sex glands working effectively — increasing virility and vitality.
- *Riboflavin (B_2)* affects the health and helps to keep the youthful appearance of your skin, nails, and hair. It also helps to prevent premature wrinkling of the facial skin as well as skin on the arms.
- *Pyridoxine (B_6)* deficiency has been known to cause impotency. B_6 can help to keep your virility at a high level despite advancing age.

LECITHIN

Lecithin is an organic phosporized fat substance, the chief constituent of brain and nerve tissues. Close to 20 percent of brain substance is made up of lecithin. Lecithin is also present in abundance in the endocrine glands, especially the gonads — both male and female. Pituitary and pineal glands contain lecithin. The pineal gland is richer in lecithin than any other part of the body. Lecithin is also an essential component of semen, and a sufficient supply is necessary for normal semen production. Lecithin has been used successfully by some doctors to treat male sexual debility and glandular exhaustion. They claim that lecithin improves virility and prevents impotency.

Lecithin can also be a great life saver by helping to prevent heart disease caused by atherosclerosis. Lecithin destroys cholesterol deposits in the arteries, thus lessening the chance of heart attack.

Dr. Lester M. Morrison, senior attending physician at Los Angeles County General Hospital, says that lecithin is "one of our most powerful weapons against disease." In the treatment of heart disease, Dr. Morrison "found lecithin to give the most rewarding results . . . " He even found that lecithin not only can prevent atherosclerosis, but in many instances, *reverse* it, making old hardened arteries younger. This is significant, since many scientists believe that "you are as young as your arteries." If lecithin can help to keep your arteries from aging, it can help you to stay younger longer.

Lecithin is truly a miraculous food supplement. It is a rich source of many rejuvenative food elements, such as vitamins E, D, and K, essential fatty acids, and especially choline and inositol, two B-vitamins that are involved in helping to prevent the aging processes. Choline and inositol are perfect fat-dissolving agents.

Lecithin should be a part of every rejuvenation diet. It is sold in all health food stores in tablet, powder, or granular form. I recommend the granular form, which is also the most economical. Two to three teaspoonfuls a day is the average dose, but some people take more.

Note: If large doses of lecithin are taken, calcium should be added to the diet (bone-meal or calcium lactate tablets) to balance the excess phosphorus obtained from the lecithin.

VITAMIN P

In the chapter on Russian Rejuvenation Secrets, I mentioned that the Russians attribute their low incidence of high blood pressure and cardiovascular diseases to their regular eating of such foods as garlic and buckwheat porridge. Russian scientists say that buckwheat supplies rutin, or vitamin P, which they have found to have a beneficial effect on the circulatory system as well as a blood pressure-reducing property.

Rutin is a bioflavonoid, a co-vitamin of ascorbic acid, or vitamin C. It increases the biological effect of vitamin C when the two are taken together, and it also has many specific beneficial properties of its own. It strengthens the blood capillaries and regulates their permeability. It also helps vitamin C to keep collagen in a healthy condition, and as I have already mentioned, collagen deterioration and the aging processes in the cardiovascular system are major causes of premature aging. Vitamin P, by preventing this deterioration, becomes an important rejuvenative factor.

BREWER'S YEAST

The single most potent rejuvenative food is brewer's yeast. Here are some of its miraculous health-building, disease-preventing and rejuvenating properties:

- It is the richest natural source of all B-vitamins, except B_{12}. As I reported previously, most of the B-vitamins — particularly B_1, B_2, B_6, B_{12}, PABA, folic acid, and pantothenic acid — are specific rejuvenators.
- It is one of the best sources of zinc, which is of specific importance for the healthy function of male sex organs and for the prevention of prostate disorders.
- It contains a huge amount of the highest quality proteins (up to 40-50% of its weight!) — 3 times more than meat. Yeast proteins are superior in quality to those in meat or many other animal sources.
- It is the richest natural source of the nucleic acids, RNA and DNA (15% of its weight!). Nucleic acids are considered to be *the* rejuvenative factor, contributing to the healthy function of all the cells in the body, and keeping the mental and physical processes at the peak of their youthful efficiency.

Brewer's yeast is available in powder form, flakes, or tablets. If consumed regularly, it can help to keep you young by preventing the degenerative diseases and halting the aging processes.

14

OPTIMUM NUTRITION —
THE TRUE FOUNTAIN OF YOUTH

I have presented to you the rejuvenation secrets from around the world — that "work". I have deliberately left out all controversial rejuvenation methods, such as cellular injections, gland and organ transplants, toxic drugs, hormones, and surgical approaches. Only those methods are reported that are 100% safe and scientifically or empirically proven.

If we summarize what has been said throughout the book so far, we will find that basically

- You are as young as your glands;
- You are as young as your cells;
- You are as young as your collagen;
- You are as young as your digestive and assimilative system;
- You are as young as your arteries;
- You are as young as your mind.

But in order to keep your glands and organs young and efficient, your digestive tract free from decay and putrefaction, your cells well oxygenated, healthy and vital, your collagen elastic, your arteries open and free from cholesterol, and your mind clear and efficient, *you have to feed your body with the highest quality nutrition* — nutrition which will supply your glands, organs, and tissues with all the *nutrients* essential for normal, healthy, and efficient functioning. So, you can see, that *the ultimate secret of staying young is basically the secret of staying healthy.* And, the secret of staying healthy is closely tied to proper nutrition. My long search for the secrets of long life leads me to the inevitable conclusion that the *True Fountain of Youth springs from optimum nutrition.* More and more researchers of the new science of Gerontology agree with me.

It is generally agreed, of course, that the state of your mind has a determining influence on your health. But even the state of your mind — your attitudes, your mental capacities and your ability to cope with severe emotional conflicts and stresses, the ability to deal with traumatic experiences or losses — depends to a great extent on the quality of your nutrition. "A sound mind can only dwell in a sound body", said the old Romans. The modern sciences of psychosomatics and nutrition have proven that the Romans were right. As Dr. Henry C. Sherman, of Columbia University, said, "not only can human life be extended, but also youthfulness can be preserved, and the extended life made more useful, by the right selection of foods." Most nutritionists are in complete agreement that chronic malnutrition is a prime cause of premature aging, and that optimum nutrition is imperative for optimum health and long life.

What constitutes OPTIMUM NUTRITION?

Now that we have agreed that optimum nutrition is absolutely necessary for the maintenance of optimum health and the prevention of disease and premature aging, the question is: *what is proper nutrition,* or *what constitutes the optimum diet for optimum health?*

If you have read more than one current book in the field of health and nutrition, you must be aware of the great confusion and disagreement among so-called "experts" and "authorities" regarding the everlasting question: *what is man's best diet for optimum health?*

There are those who believe that the so-called *"four basic food groups"* will assure optimum nutrition. There are those who advocate a *high animal protein diet,* with lots of meat. There are *vegetarians, lacto-vegetarians, lacto-ovo-vegetarians, vegans, fruitarians,* and even *breatherians,* who claim that you can get all the nutrition you need from the air you breathe although I don't know of any of them who lived long enough to prove the theory!). There are those who condemn all *seeds and grains;* those who eat seeds, *but not* grains; those who eat only vegetables that grow *above the ground;* those who condemn *honey;* and those who consider *tomatoes* and *onions* to be poisonous. There are those who advocate taking *vitamins and food supplements* — and there are those who claim that all added vitamins are harmful, and you should get all your vitamins from the food you eat. There are those who advocate eating only *raw foods,* claiming that "cooked foods are dead foods," which can only lead to premature death. Then there are those who consider the *discovery of fire* the greatest boon to man's nutrition.

Now, perhaps, you may think that I am trying to be funny — that I am exaggerating the great variety of beliefs and fads about man's proper diet. Believe me, this is just a very small sample of what is actually going on. In my capacity as a nutrition consultant, lecturer and traveler, I never cease to be amazed at the unbelievable *confusion* in this field. I have found that not only the average person, but also the well-read, well-educated veteran health seekers are thoroughly *confused* on the most vital questions related to nutrition and to the right ways and means of attaining optimum health. The more they read, the more lectures they attend — the more *confused* they become. Every book, every lecturer, and every "authority" gives them different answers and points out different roads to glorious health and long life.

I have spent three decades — a lifetime — of research to find out the *real* truth regarding optimum nutrition for optimum health. As a member of the International Society for Research on Nutrition and Diseases of Civilization, the most respected nutrition research organization in the world, which was founded by Dr. Albert Schweitzer, I have continuous access to the most up-to-date and most reliable findings regarding nutrition and its effect on man's health, which are reported by hundreds of research scientists from 75 countries. I have also traveled in many countries around the world, and have studied the eating and living habits of many natives, particularly those known for their exceptional health and longevity, as is reported in this book. On the basis of this extensive research and personal and clinical experience,

I have made my conclusions which I am sharing with you in this book. *The Airola Diet for Optimum Health and Long Life,* presented below, is not based on my own personal, subjective beliefs, likes or wishful thinking, but is based on reliable scientific sources and corroborated by overwhelming empirical and scientific evidence. This diet has not only the greatest potential for building health, preventing disease, and maintaining health, but also for preventing premature aging and keeping you younger longer.*

TEN BASIC PRINCIPLES OF OPTIMUM NUTRITION
(The Airola Diet for Optimum Health, Maximum Vitality, and Long Life)

1. **Your Optimum Diet should be made up of these three basic food groups** (in this order of importance):
   (A) Seeds, nuts, and grains
   (B) Vegetables
   (C) Fruits

Seeds, grains, and nuts are the most important and the most potent foods of all. Their nutritional value is unsurpassed by any other food. Eaten mostly raw and sprouted, but also cooked, they contain all the important nutrients essential for human growth, sustenance of health, and prevention of disease and premature aging.

All seeds and grains are beneficial, but sesame seeds, sunflower seeds, millet, buckwheat, and soybeans are especially recommended as they contain complete proteins of high biological value. All beans and peas are useful, as are all nuts. Almonds, filberts, and cashews are excellent sources of protein, as well as unsaturated fats, minerals, and other vital nutrients.

Sprouting increases the nutritional value of seeds and grains

---

* For a complete, detailed description of the AIROLA DIET FOR OPTIMUM HEALTH, see my book: *How to Get Well,* Health Plus Publishers, P.O. Box 22001, Phoenix, Arizona, 1974, 304 pages, clothbound, price $8.95. Available at all health food stores and book stores.

and makes even those grains that do not contain all the essential amino acids, into a complete protein food. Wheat, mung beans, alfalfa seeds, and soybeans make excellent sprouts.

Some grains can be eaten in cooked form. Millet, buckwheat, oats, and rice make tasty, nutritious cereals. Rye makes an excellent sourdough bread (See Chapter 3 for the value of soured lactic acid foods).

Vegetables are the next most important food in the Optimum Diet. Most vegetables contain complete proteins of high quality, plus they are an excellent source of minerals, vitamins, and enzymes. Most vegetables can be eaten raw in the form of salads. Some vegetables, such as potatoes, yams, squashes, or green beans, can be cooked. Generous use of garlic, onions, and herbs and natural spices is recommended.

Fruits, like vegetables, are excellent sources of vitamins, minerals, and enzymes. Fruits are a cleansing food. All fruits must be eaten fresh, in *season.* Out of season, some dried fruits such as raisins, prunes, figs, or apricots can be used.

Roughly, one food group should supply the bulk of each of the three meals: fruits for breakfast, seeds, nuts, or cereals for lunch, and vegetables for dinner. (See Health Menu at the end of this section.)

2. Eat mostly raw, living foods.

At least 75-80% of your diet should consist of foods in their natural, uncooked state. Numerous studies have demonstrated the superiority of raw, living foods, both for the maintenance of health and for the prevention of disease. It has been shown, for example, that you need only one-half of the amount of protein in your diet *if you eat protein foods raw instead of cooked.*

Don't be a raw-food fanatic, however. A certain amount of cooked foods (not over 20% of the total diet) will not hurt you, as it certainly does not hurt the Hunza people, who are considered to be the healthiest people in the world, with the average life expectancy of 85-90 years, and whose daily staples include such cooked foods as chapati, cereals, and soups.

If you live in an ideal tropical or subtropical climate — man's natural habitat — where fresh vegetables and fruits are available year round, you can live on raw foods almost exclusively. In colder, northern regions, a certain amount of cooked food in the form of cereals, bread, potatoes, beans, peas, etc. can be added to the diet.

3. Eat only natural foods.

Your foods should be whole, unprocessed, and unrefined, and be organically grown in fertile soil. They should preferably be grown in your own environment and eaten in *their season.*

That your health and longevity are in direct relationship to the *naturalness* of the foods you eat is a well established scientific fact. You have seen in the earlier chapters of this book that where natives eat a diet of natural, whole, unprocessed and unrefined foods, they enjoy superior health, absence of disease, and a long life. When "civilization" enters their lives in the form of denatured, refined, processed, man-made foods, disease becomes rampant among them and their life expectancy drops.

Natural foods are foods that are grown in fertile soils without chemical fertilizers and sprays, and are consumed in their *natural state,* with all the nutrients that nature put in them intact — *nothing removed and nothing added.*

4. Eat only poison-free foods.

Almost all commercially sold food today contains chemicals, either used in food producing or added during processing or packing. Some of these poisons cannot be washed out as they are *systemic,* that is, they penetrate the whole fruit or vegetable. The only solution seems to be to grow your own food, or buy certified organically grown food. Most health food stores sell such produce.

5. Complement your three basic health-building foods with the following:

A. *Milk.* The value of milk in human nutrition has been highly disputed. Some authorities claim that milk is an excellent, indeed, perfect, food for man — others insist that "milk is for calves," that it is a poison for man, causing mucus, allergies, etc.

The answer to the milk controversy is simple: milk is an

excellent health food for those whose ancestors herded dairy animals and traditionally lived on a lactose-rich diet (milk, cheese, butter). These people are genetically programmed to digest milk well, and their intestines contain plenty of the milk-digesting enzyme, *lactase*. Most white Americans of European ancestry fall into this group.

Those whose ancestors never or seldom used milk as a major element in their diets, are usually *intolerant* to milk because their intestines do not contain sufficient lactase. Most American Blacks, Chinese, Eskimos, or American Indians fall into this group. They should avoid milk completely.

The best way to use milk is in its soured form: as yogurt, kefir, acidophilus milk, or regular clabbered or butter milk. Soured milks are superior to sweet milk, as they are in a predigested form and very easily assimilated. They also help to maintain a healthy intestinal flora and prevent intestinal putrefaction and constipation. As you have seen in Chapters 1 and 4, most people known for their excellent health — Bulgarians, Swedes, Finns, Russians, and Caucasians — consume large amounts of soured milk.

Goat's or sheep's milk is superior to cow's milk as a food for humans. Homemade cottage cheese, some natural cheese, and a certain amount of butter can be added to the diet.

B. *Cold-pressed vegetable oils.* High quality, fresh, cold-pressed, crude and unrefined vegetable oils are recommended as an addition to the diet. The average daily amount is 2 tablespoons.

Make sure oils are genuinely *cold-pressed,* and fresh, *not rancid.* Most oils, even those sold in health food stores, are *not* cold-pressed, even when the label says they are. The only oils that would be likely to be the real cold-pressed oils, would be olive oil (especially imported Italian or Spanish oil in metal cans) or sesame seed oil.

C. *Honey.* Natural, raw, unheated, unfiltered, and unprocessed honey is the only sweetener allowed in the AIROLA OPTIMUM DIET. Honey possesses miraculous nutritional and medicinal properties. As I have mentioned in previous chapters, most centenarians in Russia, Bulgaria, and Abkhazia use honey liberally in their diets.

Honey is especially beneficial in the diets of older people and children. It increases calcium retention in the system, helps to prevent nutritional anemia, and is beneficial in heart, kidney, and liver disorders, colds, poor circulation, and complexion problems.

D. *Speical protective foods.* The optimum diet should include the following special protective and super-nutritious foods: brewer's yeast (3-5 tbsp. a day), kelp (2-3 tablets or 1 tsp. of granules), wheat germ (only if available fresh — not more than one week old after it is made — 2-3 tbsp. a day) and fish liver oil (1 tbsp. a day — only in colder climates, during winter months).

E. *Natural vitamin and mineral supplements.* As effective insurance against nutritional deficiencies and protection against the harmful effects of our increasingly toxic environment and toxic residues in natural foods, take good quality natural vitamin and mineral supplements regularly. When planning a specific rejuvenation program, take all the vitamins mentioned in Chapter 13 of this book.

6. Avoid an excess of protein in your diet.

The optimum diet of three basic foods — seeds, nuts and grains; vegetables; and fruits — supplemented with the special super-foods and food supplements named above, will assure you an adequate supply of all required nutrients for optimum health and long life, *including sufficient amounts of complete high quality proteins.* A moderate amount of eggs, fish, or meat may be added to this basic diet, if desired — particularly fish in coastal areas, or meat in far northern regions with long winters, *but their inclusion is not necessary.* In temperate, sub-tropical or tropical climates, the highest level of health and longevity can be best achieved and maintained without meat.

A high animal protein diet is definitely detrimental to health and may cause or contribute to the development of many of our most common diseases, such as arthritis, heart disease, cancer, osteoporosis, schizophrenia, kidney damage, vitamin and mineral deficiencies, etc., as proven in extensive clinical studies. A high protein diet also causes premature aging and lowers life expectancy. (Well-documented evidence regarding the dangers of a high protein diet can be found in my books, *Are You Confused?* and *How to Get Well.* Also, see Chapter 8 in this book.)

7. Drink pure, natural water.

The best water for drinking is pure, natural, uncontaminated spring, river, or well water. Avoid prolonged drinking of distilled water. Dozens of actual studies from the United States, England, Europe, and Japan, show that the minerals in naturally hard water are important to man's nutrition. Studies show that where people drink naturally hard (highly mineralized) water, they have less heart disease, less tooth decay, less diabetes, and less arteriosclerosis. Minerals, as they are naturally present in drinking water, have been an essential part of man's mineral nutrition since the beginning of his life on this planet.

Contrary to what some "experts" claim, inorganic minerals in natural water *are* effectively absorbed and utilized in human metabolism. We need both organic and inorganic minerals. Foods supply organic minerals, and water inorganic minerals (See Chapters 3 and 8).

8. Cleanse your system periodically with juice fasting.

One of the main reasons for most diseases and premature aging is disordered metabolism and the consequent retention of waste matter in the cells and tissues of the body — or what is medically known as *autotoxemia.* Juice fasting (see Chapter 3) is the best and safest way to cleanse the body of the accumulated toxins and restore and normalize all the vital functions.

Always keeping your body clean internally and in the best working condition is the best way to prevent premature aging. You should fast at least 1 week to 10 days each year, preferably in the spring. Actual studies showed that animals who fasted periodically lived 2½ to 5 times longer than animals who always ate as much as they wanted.

(For complete details on *Why, How, and When to Fast,* see my book. *How to Keep Slim, Healthy, and Young with JUICE FASTING.* Also, see Chapter 3 of this book.)

9. **Cultivate the following health-promoting eating habits:**
   a. Eat only when really hungry.
   b. Eat slowly and in a relaxed atmosphere.
   c. Eat several small meals during the day in preference to a few large meals.
   d. Do not mix too many foods at the same meal — the less mixing, the better the digestion.
   e. Do not mix raw fruits and raw vegetables at the same meal — they are incompatible in regard to enzymes, and mixing them will only result in poor digestion.
   f. When protein-rich foods are eaten with other foods, eat the protein-rich foods first. It is wrong to eat a large vegetable salad in the beginning of the meal, and then continue with meat or other protein food. For proper digestion, protein requires lots of hydrochloric acid, which is more plentiful in the beginning of the meal when the stomach is empty.
   g. Finally, practice *systematic undereating*. Systematic undereating is the number one health and longevity secret. Studies of centenarians around the world show that they are moderate eaters throughout their lives. You never see an obese centenarian. Overeating, on the other hand, is one of the main causes of disease and premature aging. Overeating and particularly overindulgence in proteins, is especially dangerous to older people who are less active and have a slowed metabolism. The unbelievable fact is that the less you eat, the less hungry you feel, because the food will be more efficiently digested and better utilized.
   At a recent symposium on the relationship between nutrition and longevity, a highly competent group of international experts in the field agreed that the restriction of food intake, to a point that would be considered undernutrition by contemporary standards, both lengthens the life and improves the health by reducing the susceptibility to the diseases of aging (Journal of Clinical Nutrition, August, 1972).
   As Benjamin Franklin said, "To lengthen thy life, lessen thy meals." My own aphorism on the subject goes

as follows: "A man's belt length is his life's length . . . *in reverse:* the longer the belt — the shorter the life."

10. Avoid the following health destroyers:

This is the list of *do nots,* the things you must avoid if you wish to achieve optimum health. All these factors are scientifically well-proven to be potent health and longevity destroyers.

- All tobacco.. Smoking is also a potent complexion destroyer. I can spot any woman who has smoked 5 years or longer just by looking at her complexion, which always acquires a dull, lifeless, coarse, masculine, and wrinkled look.
- Coffee, tea, chocolate, cola drinks, and other soft drinks.
- Excessive use of salt.
- Excessive consumption of alcohol.
- Harmful spices: black and white pepper, mustard, white vinegar.
- White sugar and white flour, and everything made with them.
- All processed, refined, canned, or factory-made foods.
- All rancid foods, such as rancid seeds, nuts, oils, and old, rancid wheat germ. (Any wheat germ is rancid if it is older than one week after it is made.)
- All chemical drugs, except in emergencies, ordered by a doctor.
- All household and environmental toxic chemicals: garden sprays; air fresheners; household chemicals and cleaners; detergents (use soap flakes); hair sparys; chemically cleaned or treated clothes, beds, or wallpaper; bug and fly killers; etc.
- Avoid a sedentary life and lack of exercise and relaxation.

The last point I would like to elaborate upon a bit.

Today's sedentary living is one of the main causes of our physical degeneration. Medical evidence to the effect that ample, *regular* exercise is imperative for optimum health and long life is overwhelming. Lack of sufficient exercise contributes to the development of many of our most killing diseases, and is one of the main causes of nearly one million deaths a year from heart attacks in the United States.

The best form of exercise is regular walking — an hour or two a day.

Speaking of walking reminds me of a story:

A man who lived to be 100 years old was asked: "What is your secret of long life?"

"Walking . . . . daily walking," the man replied. "You see, when my wife and I were married, we agreed that every time we had an argument, I'd take a walk outdoors. And for the past 80 years, I've been outdoors walking most of the time."

Relaxation and peace of mind — these are two other vital health factors that are missing in modern man's life. Emotional and mental stresses such as fears, anxiety, worries, tensions, depressions, hate, jealousy, unhappiness, deprivation of love, and loneliness, can cause practically every disease in the medical dictionary, and thereby shorten life.

Relaxation, peace of mind, a positive outlook on life, a contented spirit, an absence of envy and jealousy, a cheerful disposition, love of mankind, and faith in God — these are all powerful health-promoting factors without which optimum health cannot be achieved.

YOUR HEALTH MENU

Based on the information presented in this chapter, your daily menu for a health-building and rejuvenating diet should look something like this:

UPON ARISING: Glass of pure water — plain, or with choice of freshly squeezed citrus juice: ½ lime, ¼ lemon, ½ grapefruit, or one orange to a glass of water.

OR: Large cup of warm herb tea sweetened with honey. Choice of rose hips, peppermint, camomile, or any of your favorite herbs.

OR: Glass of freshly made fruit juice from any available fruit or berry in season: apple, pineapple, orange, cherry, pear, etc. The juice should be diluted with water, half and half. No canned or frozen juices — the juice must be freshly made just before drinking.

After this morning drink, you should walk for one hour in the fresh air, combining your walk with deep-breathing exercises and all the calisthenics you can manage to squeeze in. If you have a garden, or if you live on a farm, you should get in a couple of hours of hard physical labor.

Upon returning from your long walk, or garden work, and after a cold shower to wash the perspiration away, you are now, *but not before,* ready for your breakfast.

BREAKFAST: Fresh fruits, preferably organically grown: apple, orange, banana, grapes, grapefruit, or any available berries and fruits, *in season.* Cup of yogurt, kefir, or homemade soured milk, preferably goat's milk (see Chapter 3 for recipes and instructions). Handful of raw nuts, such as almonds, cashews, peanuts. or sesame seeds. Nuts and seeds can be crushed or ground in your own seed grinder (sold in health food stores) and sprinkled over yogurt. ½ cup of homemade cottage cheese.

OR: Large bowl of fresh Fruit Salad á lá Airola (see instructions at the end of this Chapter).

OR: Bowl of rolled oats, uncooked, with 4-6 soaked prunes, or 2-3 figs, and a handful of unsulfured raisins. Glass of raw unpasteurized milk, perferably goat's milk, or yogurt.

OR: Bowl of sprouted wheat or other sprouted seeds with yogurt and/or available fresh fruits.

MIDMORNING SNACK: One apple, banana, or other fruit.

LUNCH: Bowl of whole-grain cereal, such as millet cereal, buckwheat cereal, or Kruska. Any other available whole-grain cereals, such as oats, barley, rice, or corn, can be used. Dry milk powder (non-instant kind) can be added to the water when cereals are cooked. Large glass of raw milk, preferably goat's milk. One tablespoon of cold-pressed vegetable oil and/or one tablespoon of honey can be used on cereal.

OR: Large bowl of fresh Fruit Salad á lá Airola (if not eaten for breakfast).

OR: Bowl of freshly prepared vegetable soup or any other cooked vegetable dish, such as potatoes, yams, squash, beans and corn tortillas. Kelp, sea salt, cold-pressed vegetable oil, and fresh butter, as well as any of the natural herbs can be used for seasoning. Glass of yogurt or other soured milk.

1 - 2 slices of whole-grain bread, preferably sour-dough rye bread (see Chapter 2), 1 or 2 slices of natural cheese (available at health food stores). Never use processed cheeses.

MID AFTERNOON:

Glass of fresh fruit or vegetable juice.

OR: Cup of your favorite herb tea, sweetened with honey.

OR: One apple, banana, pear, or other available fruit.

DINNER: Large bowl of fresh, green vegetable salad. Use any and all available vegetables — preferably those in season — including tomatoes, avocados, and all available sprouts, such as alfalfa seed sprouts, mung bean sprouts, etc. Carrots, shredded red beets, and onion should be staples in every salad. Garlic, if your social life permits. Salad should be attractively prepared and served with homemade dressing of lemon juice (or apple cider vinegar) and cold-pressed vegetable oil, seasoned with herbs, garlic powder, a little sea salt, cayenne pepper, etc.

But all vegetables can be also placed attractively on the plate without mixing them into a salad, and eaten one at a time — this is, by far, the superior way of eating vegetables.

2 or 3 middle sized boiled or baked potatoes in jackets. Prepared cooked vegetable course, if desired: eggplant, artichoke, sweet potatoes, yams, squash, or other vegetables. Use kelp powder or sea salt sparingly for seasoning; also any or all of the usual garden herbs. Fresh homemade cottage cheese, or 1 - 2 slices of natural cheese.

Fresh butter or 1 tbsp. of cold-pressed vegetable oil (can be used on salad, soup, or potatoes).

Glass of yogurt or other soured milk.

OR: Any of the recommended lunch choices, if fresh vegetable salad is eaten at lunch.

BEDTIME SNACK:
Glass of fresh milk, or nut-milk, or seed-milk (made in electric liquifier from raw seeds or raw nuts and water — milk can be added or not, according to preference) with a tablespoon of honey.

OR: Glass of yogurt with brewer's yeast.

OR: Cup of your favorite herb tea with a slice of whole grain bread with butter and a slice of natural cheese.

OR: One apple.

Vital points to remember
1. The above menu is only a very general outline — a skeleton, around which an individual diet for optimum nutri-

tion should be built. It can be followed as it is, of course — I know of thousands of people who live on such a diet and enjoy extraordinary health. But it also can be modified and changed to adapt to your specific requirements and conditions, your country's customs, your climate, the availability of foods, your health condition, your preferences, etc.

2. Whatever changes you make, however, keep in mind that the bulk of your diet should consist of seeds, nuts, and grains, and fresh vegetables and fruits, preferably organically grown, and up to 80% of them eaten raw. Eat as great a variety of available foods as possible, but not in the same meal, of course. Do not shun potatoes and avocados and bananas because you think they are fattening — they are not!

3. The menu for lunch and dinner is interchangeable. One big vegetable meal should be eaten at least once a day. If it is eaten for lunch, some of the lunch suggestions can be eaten for dinner.

4. Remember, when you eat protein-rich foods (cottage cheese, nuts, beans, etc.) together with carbohydrate-rich foods (salads, fruits, etc.) — eat the protein-rich foods *first*, or *together with* carbohydrate-rich foods, but *not after*. If you follow this advice, your digestion will improve dramatically.

5. Do not drink water with meals. If thirsty, drink between meals, or 15 minutes before meals. Milk and yogurt are foods.

6. If you are taking vitamins and other food supplements, take them *with* meals.

7. One or two tablespoons of brewer's yeast should be taken either with breakfast or lunch, or between meals with fruit juice or yogurt.

8. Finally, if you follow this Health Menu *every day of your life,* you can live a long life and enjoy the highest possible level of health. And be assured that this Airola Optimum Diet will supply you not only with *all* the vitamins, minerals, essential fatty acids, trace elements, enzymes and the other identified and unidentified nutritive substances, but also with an adequate amount of the highest quality proteins you need for optimum health!

Fruit Salad á lá Airola

1 bowl fresh fruits, organically grown if possible
1 handful raw nuts and/or sunflower seeds
3-4 soaked prunes or handful of raisins, unsulfured
3 tbsp. cottage cheese, preferably homemade, unsalted
1 tbsp. raw wheat germ (only if available absolutely fresh, not more than a week old)
3 tbsp. yogurt
1 tbsp. wheat germ oil (only if 100% fresh, not rancid — if not available, replace with olive or sesame oil)
2 tsp. natural, unpasteurized honey
1 tsp. fresh lemon juice

Wash all fruits carefully, and dry. Use any available fruits and berries, but try to get at least three or four different kinds. Peaches, grapes, pears, papaya, bananas, strawberries, and fresh pineapple are particularly good for producing a delightful bouquet of rich, penetrating flavors. A variety of colors will make the salad festive and attractive to the eye.

Chop or slice bigger fruits, but leave grapes and berries whole. Place them in a large bowl and add prunes and nuts (nuts and sunflower seeds could be crushed). Make a dressing with one teaspoon honey (or more if most of the fruits used are sour), one teaspoon of lemon juice, and two tablespoons of water. Pour over the fruit, add wheat germ, and toss well. Mix cottage cheese, yogurt, wheat germ oil, and one teaspoon of honey in a separate cup until it is fairly smooth in texture and pour it on top of the salad. Sprinkle with nuts and sunflower seeds. Serve at once.

This is not only a most delicious dish, but it is the most nutritious and perfectly balanced meal I know. It is a storehouse of high-grade proteins and all the essential vitamins, minerals, fatty acids and enzymes you need for optimum health. This salad should be a daily *must* for the rejuvenation-conscious and health-conscious alike.

15

CENTENARIANS SPEAK . . .

Observations, clinical tests, vital statistics, animal studies, laboratory experiments, theories — all these are useful when we are trying to determine the secrets of long life. But nothing is as convincing as personal testimony of those who have achieved the enviable age of 100 or more years. Let's hear from some of them, in their own words, their secrets of superior health and a long life of youthful vitality.

While in Russia, I met several centenarians. I discovered that they all had a few things in common: they all were moderate eaters; almost all of them used lots of honey in their diets; they all were either vegetarians or ate only very little meat; they all were slim; and they all were happy!

One man, 126 years old, told me:

"I've worked hard all of my life, but never had much money to worry about. I walk at least 5 miles every day, and ride a horse. I eat very little, and only when hungry — I never eat at regular times, but just when I feel really hungry. I was married four times, each time to a younger wife. Maybe this has helped me to stay young!"

The Russian Minister of Health told a story of a Russian centenarian from Caucasus who lived to the respectable age of 146 years. When asked for the reasons for his enviable longevity, the man said:

"I've never had a boss over me. I have never been envious of what others have. And I have periodically rejuvenated myself by marrying three times!"

The above two cases seem to demonstrate that vibrant health, long life, and sexual virility go hand in hand. Dr.

Bernard Jensen, who has studied the lives of centenarians in Russia, Turkey, and Bulgaria, made a similar observation. Upon his return, he said:

"I've made a remarkable observation: almost all centenarians I've met have been married several times."

My conclusion is that we do not stop sexual activity because we grow old — we grow old because we stop sexual activity.

Recently, while making up an electoral list, Turkish authorities found the oldest man in Turkey, a 144 year old farmer, Mustafa Tasci. He remarried at 83, when his first wife died, and he has 13 children and 50 grandchildren. Tasci is a vegetarian — he has never eaten meat in his life. He does not smoke, and has never drunk alcohol. He walks a mile and a half each day, and he still works in his orchard.

Mustafa Tasci's secret of long life is summed up in his words:

"Eat moderately; stay away from meat, smoke, and alcohol; work every day; and surround yourself with young children."

The oldest man in the world today is Shirali Mislimov. He is 166 years of age and lives in the Russian province of Azerbaidzhan, in the Caucasian mountains. Mislimov's formula for a long and happy life includes: clean air, natural foods, a slow pace, a kind heart, and a lot of work.

Here's his secret of long life in his own words, delivered in the poetic language of the Azerbaidzhan mountains:

"I was never in a hurry in my life, and I'm in no hurry to die now."

"There are two sources of long life:"

"One is a gift of nature, and it is the pure air and clear water of the mountains, the fruit of the earth, peace, rest, and the soft warm climate of the highlands."

"The second source is within us. He lives long who enjoys life and who bears no jealousy of others, whose heart harbors no malice or anger, who sings a lot and cries a little, who rises and retires with the sun, who likes to work, and who knows how to rest."

Regarding his diet, the 166-year-old Mislimov said: "I eat the usual food our people here have been eating for generations: mostly fruits and homemade cheeses, and a very little meat. And I drink a little tea. I never eat when I am not hungry," he concluded.

One of the most inspiring examples of a long, happy, and useful life is the story of a Venetian nobleman of the 16th century, Luigi Cornaro.

A physical wreck, facing invalidism and death at the age of 36, rejected by contemporary doctors as incurable, he took his health into his own hands and began reading, studying, and experimenting in order to save his life. In a few years, he achieved a robust and glowing health, and lived a happy and useful life in full possession of his physical and mental capacities, to the age of 103.

Luigi Cornaro wrote a book to tell others of his secrets of bouyant health and long life, called, *A Sure and Certain Method for Attaining a Long and Healthy Life.* The title of the recent edition is, *The Art of Living Long.*

One of Cornaro's secrets is: "Not to satiate oneself with food is the science of health." He discovered that systematic undereating, or moderate eating, was the secret of feeling great. "My greatest discovery was that the less I ate, the better I felt," said Luigi Cornaro.

Carefully selecting his foods, he discovered that he felt best by eating grains, mostly in the form of bread, although he did use some animal foods in moderation.

He also discovered that diet alone was not sufficient to assure the highest level of health — that the influence of the mind and emotions had an important role to play in the overall health picture.

"I have also," he wrote, "preserved myself, as far as I have been able, from those other disorders from which it is more difficult to be exempt: I mean melancholy, hatred, and the other passions of the soul, which all appear greatly to affect the body."

In chapter 11, I told you about the renowned Chinese professor and herbalist, Li Chung Yun, who lived to be 256 years old. Researchers and writers who studied his life in detail, attributed his long life to his vegetarian diet and special rejuvenative herb teas which he drank all of his life: ginseng and gotu-kola.

Li Chung Yun himself, however, had a different idea for the reason of his long life. When asked to what he attributed his long life, he said:

"I attribute my long life to INWARD CALM".

In all my studies of people who lived extraordinarily long lives in various parts of the world, I have found that in addition to all the other factors, such as sound nutrition of simple, unadulterated foods, scanty eating, poison free environment, and plenty of exercise, they all possessed that unmistakable quality Professor Yun was talking about — *INWARD CALM.* They were contented, happy with their lot, didn't envy anyone, and they usually held important positions in the community and were respected by their families, neighbors, and the other villagers. This sense of importance, of being useful, having the respect and adoration of families and neighbors is, in my opinion, an extremely important factor in longevity. Unfortunately, in the United States, oldsters usually face the opposite lot: they are excluded from a useful role in society, shoved into old peoples' homes, forgotten by families and relatives; they feel isolated, useless, and unrespected.

Dr. Alexander Leaf, chief of medical services at Massachusetts General Hospital in Boston, made an extensive study in three sections of the world where people live extraordinarily long lives: The Andean village of Vilcabamba, Ecuador; the Hunza Kingdom in Kashmir; and the Black Sea coastal area of Abkhazia, in Russia.

In Abkhazia, Dr. Leaf met a 130-year old woman who held the title of the fastest tea leaf picker on the collective farm where she worked.

In Hunza, he found a 110-year old man who did a full day's work in the fields among younger men, binding hay on a steep hillside.

In Vilcabamba, he interviewed a 123-year old man who had retired as a hunter 50 years ago, and now was actively engaged in farming.

All of these people were in excellent physical condition. Dr. Leaf's conclusion was that regular physical exercise, heredity, and a sense of importance, in addition to their generally low-calorie and low-protein diets, were important keys to a longer life.

I can still picture in my mind a 104-year old man I met on one of my trips to Russia. He was living in a tiny mountainous village in Abkhazia and was herding sheep from horseback. At 104, he was still a superb horseman, able to mount his horse more easily than a typical American teenager could. When I asked him to what he attributed his long life, he said:

"I've had 3 wives, I have 17 children, 48 grandchildren, and many great and great-great-grandchildren. I am loved and respected by all of them, and I have much to live for. I have never had many possessions. I always worked for others, and I have never been jealous of what others have. I go to sleep with the sun, and get up with the sun. I eat simple things, and only when I am really hungry. I never smoked, and I taste a little wine on festive occasions. I love these mountains, and the sheep, and my horse, and I sing throughout most of the day. Life is wonderful when you can enjoy good health . . . "

An American centenarian, Thomas Dayton, 107 years old, expressed his secret of long life thus:

"I kept my body active, but my mind at rest. People worry too much . . . I've always taken care of myself physically, as well as mentally, by eating regular meals and getting plenty of sleep. I eat a lot of fruit — mostly apples, pears, and peaches. I drink goat's milk, because if has more nourishment than cow's milk, And I have never smoked."

Thomas Dayton married his second wife when he was 73.

I would like to conclude this chapter with the statement made by Dr. Alexander Leaf, M.D., who traveled to Hunza, Caucasus, Abkhazia, and Vilcabamba, to study the lifestyles of the centenarians and determine the causes of their exceptional longevity. Dr. Leaf says:

"I returned from my travels convinced that vigorous, active old age, free from debility and senility, is possible." *(Nutrition Today,* Vol. 8, Number 5, October/November, 1973.)

My own studies made in the same parts of the world that Dr. Leaf studied, as well as in other, less known or accessible areas, confirm Dr. Leaf's conclusion. The phenomenon of longevity seems to have many causes. But the most prominent contributing causes to long life seem to be:

1. Adequate nutrition provided by a simple diet of natural foods.
2. Low-calorie, low-fat, low-protein diet.
3. Plenty of exercise or outdoor work.
4. A certain genetic influence — centenarians usually had parents who likewise attained great age.
5. A positive, peaceful state of mind, or as 256-year old Li Chung Yun put it, *Inward calm.*

16

ARE YOU
SHORTENING YOUR LIFE?

There are many ways of prolonging life, as we have seen so far. There are many secrets of looking and feeling young, secrets that "work", and secrets that don't. As one cynic said, "The best method of looking young is to lie about your age." There are quite a few famous health and long life experts who are doing just that. It always impresses the audiences when a speaker says, "Look at me, I am 82 years young!" How would they know that his birth certificate shows only 72?

By far the best method of prolonging life and looking and feeling young was expressed by Herbert Spencer, when he wrote:

"The whole secret of prolonging one's life consists in doing nothing to shorten it."

Dr. A. Ochsner, noted authority on aging, reported in the *Journal of American Geriatrics Society,* that premature senility can be controlled to a great extent *by avoiding factors that accelerate aging.*

If we would live in accordance with all the known laws of health, and *do nothing to cause disease and shorten life,* we would live to be at least 150 years of age, and enjoy youthful vitality, including sexual virility, throughout life. But man seems to go out of his way, using his ingenuity and inventiveness, to ruin his health and shorten his life. He is the only creature that spoils his food before he eats it − by heating, frying, freezing, preserving, processing, and refining. He poisons his air and water supply. He depletes his soil by chemicals that grow nutritionally inferior food which cannot sustain health. He ignores the basic laws of all life — need for motion — and shortens his life by a sedentary way of living, without sufficient physical exertion. Relaxation and peace of mind are most important for health and long life, but his life is filled with continuous stresses because he is haunted by the insatiable drive for more material wealth and power. He digs his own grave with his knife and fork, eating denatured, overprocessed, nutritionless, and poisoned foods which can result in most of the serious or fatal deseases such as cancer, arthritis, heart disease, etc.

Man, indeed, seems to do all he can do to shorten his life!

Are you shortening *your* life?

I must admit that we are all subjected to certain health-destroying factors that we cannot avoid. In this age of universal chemical pollution, it is not easy to live so that our health will not be endangered. Smog is difficult to escape. Equally difficult to escape are the thousands of health-destroying and life-shortening poisons in water and food. But a few things can be done to improve our individual lives and to protect our health to the greatest possible extent.

I must tell you a true story that happened recently — an example of how some people shorten their lives, largely by ignorance.

A couple in their middle years came to me for nutritional consultation. He was a balding, overweight man, looking to be around 60. She was the opposite: thin, emaciated, with a dull complexion and graying hair, appearing to be in her early fifties. I had my first surprise when I found that he was 46 and she was 39!

The couple told me that they were at the end of their rope; they were desperate for help. Some readers of my books directed them to me. This is the kind of people a nutritionist usually sees — first they try everything else — medical specialists, expensive tests, fancy clinics, countless drugs, psychiatrists, more medical specialists — without receiving any help. Then they are ready, as a last-ditch attemp, to go to a nutritionist.

Here is their story, in his words:

"We had pretty good health until a few years ago. But

then something happened. My wife became tired all the time, lost all of her interest in life — just laid in bed all day, complaining of aches and pains. Doctors couldn't find out what was wrong with her. They gave her hormone shots, suspecting hypothyroidism and premature menopause. But nothing helped. I began putting on weight a few years ago. I'm tired all the time, hardly able to drag my legs. I can't sleep. Our sex life is completely finished, too — I haven't touched my wife for a year. Not that she cares — she is so beat that sex is the farthest thing from her mind. I'm afraid of losing my job — I can't think straight, and I bark at everyone at work. I have a responsible executive position in my company and it's getting to be too much for me. After a few hours at the office, I'm ready to quit and go home. Coffee is the only thing that keeps me going. I drink a cup about every half hour."

As he talked, they both chain smoked. The interview revealed that this couple had been violating all of the known rules of health for decades. Both were heavy smokers and heavy drinkers. Their life was centered around almost nightly parties where they drank a lot of alcohol. Their diet consisted largely of coffee — at least 10-15 cups a day — varied snacks, frozen dinners, sweets, and party snacks at night. They hardly ever ate fresh vegetables or fruits, nor whole grain bread or cereals. They drank no milk, but ate plenty of ice cream, and consumed lots of soft drinks. Their physical exercise was limited to walking from the bed to the bar, and walking to and from the car. They even used a push button to change the channels on the television. It is significant that *none of the doctors they visited had ever asked them what they ate or how they lived.*

When I suggested to them that their premature aging — her premature menopause, run-down condition, and gray hair; his obesity, lack of vitality, and sexual impotence — was brought about by their terrible living habits, their total disregard of all the elementary rules of health, they looked not only surprised, but disappointed. They expected that I would give them a bottle of vitamin pills which would miraculously wipe out all their problems and restore their health and youth. Instead, I said that if they wanted their health and youth back, their libido and vitality restored, they must stop smoking, stop drinking alcohol, soft drinks, and coffee, and stop eating nutritionless junk foods. They must give up all-night parties and start regular strenuous physical exercise such as walking and jogging. They must begin eating health-building foods instead of health-destroying foods. In addition, I promised to outline for them a comprehensive revitalization and rejuvenation program with a special diet of health-building foods and special vitamins and food supplements.

It was difficult to convince them to make such a drastic change in their lifestyle. It had never occured to them — and no doctor had ever suggested — that their conditions had anything to do with their way of living. But, they had no choice: life was so miserable that they were willing to try anything.

Their program started with a short cleansing fast. Then a complete and rigid program of exercise, rest, and a diet of optimum nutrition — plenty of fresh vegetables and fruits, whole grain cereals, seeds and nuts, yogurt, honey, cold-pressed vegetable oils. No meat; no canned or processed foods; no white sugar or white bread; no sweets, ice cream, donuts, or soft drinks. They agreed to stop drinking alcohol completely, and to try to stop smoking.

It took three months for results to begin to show. It took another three months before they could stop smoking. After six months, they reported to me that my program had "accomplished a miracle": they felt like new people! All tiredness was gone, her hair began to turn darker, menstrual irregularity disappeared, and she was full of vitality and slept like a baby. He lost over 30 pounds, he enjoyed his work at the office once more, and their sex life was completely straightened out. I've never seen a happier or more enthusiastic couple.

Are you shortening your life?

If you are, the true story I've just told you shows that you can make your life over, you can stop killing yourself and start growing younger! This book can show you the way. Turn the pages back and reread Chapter 14. Follow the rejuvenative and health-building optimum diet I gave you, and avoid all the health destroyers and life shorteners I listed at the end of that chapter. If you will do these things, I assure you that good things will begin to happen in your life: you will feel better; you will sleep better; you will lose those extra pounds you're carrying around; you will enjoy life more; you will ignore and overlook the inevitable daily irritations that used to drive you mad; you will have a new surge of vitality, and if you have been losing interest in sex, you will experience new virility and libido that you have not known since your honeymoon!

How do I know that these things will happen to you? Simple: I have thousands of letters in my files from readers of my books and those for whom I have planned a personalized nutritional program — they all report miraculous changes in their lives after changing their living habits. This works by the simple natural law of cause and effect. You have been violating the basic laws of health, and you have been feeling accordingly. You cannot fool Mother Nature. "Whatsoever ye sow, that also shall ye reap". Stop working *against nature* and start working *with nature*. Give nature a chance! Your body has a remarkable regenerative capacity. Remove all the health-destroyers and life shorteners from your life — smoking, drinking, white sugar and white flour, processed, refined, and de-natured and poisoned foods, drugs, and other chemicals — and follow the rejuvenation diet described in Chapter 14. Make use of all the various health and rejuvenation secrets from around the world which you have learned from this book, and *you will be amazed at the results!* You will begin to *grow younger* instead of growing older. Not only will most of your present health problems be solved, but you will feel and act like a new person. You will enjoy peace, contentment, happiness, and joy in living as you never have before.

Are you shortening your life and growing old prematurely?

You can change your life pattern and start growing younger — TODAY! Today is the beginning of the rest of your life. You may continue in the old rut, and grow older by the day — or you may change over and begin a new way of life which will help you to grow younger in body, mind, and spirit. It's up to you!

Conclusion

WHY LIVE LONG?

It is hardly worth-while to learn how to live long if you have to live a life of suffering from one agonizing disease after another. A long life makes sense only if it can be lived in vibrant health, and enjoyed in the active, productive pursuit of one's most treasured interests.

Unfortunately, there are very few people around who are really enjoying perfect health. Most are sick, semi-sick, or half-healthy. Really healthy persons have become so rare that the standards of good health are no longer very high. One man, whom I tried to admonish to stop smoking, said to me, "Why should I? I am perfectly healthy. Smoking hasn't ruined my health!" Yet, he consumes a handful of pills each day — aspirins for his headaches, alkalizers for his indigestion, laxatives, tranquilizers, and sleeping aids. He was in the hospital twice during the last year, he has high blood pressure, and wears dentures at the age of 38. "Perfectly healthy," indeed!

Many feel that if they are still standing on their feet and are not confined to a hospital bed, they are in "good health." But a study conducted by Tulane University in Louisiana, showed that 92% of all Americans — 92 out of every 100! — have something wrong with them, and are suffering from some form of physical or mental disorders!

No wonder I so often hear the following comment, especially when I lecture to groups not previously exposed to health-building ideas:

"Why should I stop enjoying such fruits of civilization as alcohol, tobacco, and gourmet foods I like — only to be assured of a few more years of life? I'd rather enjoy eating, drinking, and doing what I like, and die a few years earlier!"

I wish to stress two things:

First, if eating and doing "what you like" destroys your health and ages you prematurely, then it defeats its purpose, because you can hardly *enjoy* living if you are not healthy.

Second, the reason for changing your health-destroying eating and living habits is not to live a few more years, but *to live whatever years you are going to live in bouyant health – and ENJOYING THEM.*

Moreover, the real purpose of attaining better physical health and a longer life is not just the mere enjoyment of life, but a higher, divine purpose for which life was given to us. All endeavors toward attaining better health and extended longevity would be a wasted effort unless the healthy body is used as a worthy temple for the spirit to dwell in and develop. The purpose of our lives is not just the building of magnificent bodies, or living a long time, but perfecting and refining our divine spirits, and becoming more God-like. "Be ye perfect, even as your Father, which is in heaven, is perfect", said the Man from Nazareth. Our life on this planet, at this time in history, is just a short episode in the eternal divine plan of human development – a schooling period aimed at improving and perfecting our human and divine characteristics. Only those who are unaware of the high goal and divine purpose of human life talk about "eat, drink, and be merry."

Although this book deals with material and physical aspects of attaining an optimum level of health and a long life, we wish to emphasize the divine nature and purpose of all life, and that the real purpose of achieving good health is to prepare a way for our spiritual growth and perfection. Freed from disease and pain, we will be able to pursue our true purpose in life – the perfection of our human and divine characteristics and the refinement of our spirit.

With these words, I dedicate this book *TO YOU,* sincerely hoping that it will not only help to improve your health and rejuvenate your body and mind, but also bring more happiness and purpose into your life.

INDEX

ABOUT THE AUTHOR

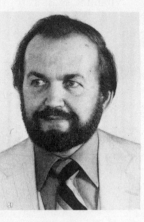

Paavo Airola, Ph.D., N.D., is an internationally recognized nutritionist, naturopathic physician, lecturer, and an award-winning author. He studied nutrition, biochemistry, and biological medicine in Europe and spent many years of research and study in European biological clinics and research centers. He is considered to be the leading authority on biological medicine and wholistic approach to healing in the United States. He lectures extensively, and worldwide, both to professionals and laymen, holding yearly educational seminars for physicians. He has recently lectured at the Stanford University Medical School.

Dr. Airola is the author of eleven widely-read books, notably his two international best-sellers, *Are You Confused?* and *How To Get Well.* The American Academy of Public Affairs issued Dr. Airola the Award of Merit for his book, *There Is A Cure For Arthritis. Are You Confused?* is heralded by many nutritionists, doctors, and critics as "the most important health book ever published," "a must reading for every sincere health seeker."

His comprehensive handbook on natural healing, *How To Get Well,* is the most authoritative and practical manual on biological medicine in print. It outlines complete nutritional, herbal, and other alternative biological therapies for all of our most common ailments and is used as a textbook in several universities and medical schools. It is regarded as a reliable reference manual by doctors, researchers, nutritionists, and students of health, nutrition, and biological medicine.

Dr. Airola's newest book, *Hypoglycemia: A Better Approach,* has revolutionized the concept of and the therapeutic approach to this insidious, complex, and devastating affliction which has assumed epidemic proportions.

Dr. Airola is President of the International Academy of Biological Medicine; a member of the International Naturopathic Association; and a member of the International Society for Research on Civilization Diseases and Environment, the prestigious forum for world-wide research, founded by Dr. Albert Schweitzer. He is listed in *The Directory of International Biography, The Blue Book, The Men of Achievement, Who's Who In American Art,* and *Who's Who in the West.*